PREVENTIVE & SOCIAL MEDICINE

B. Jain's B.H.M.S. SOLVED PAPERS

PREVENTIVE & SOCIAL MEDICINE

Write or visit for books

PRABHUS BOOKS
(A House of Books of your choice)
Ayurveda College Jn.,
Old Sreekanteswaram Road,
Thiruvananthapuram - 695 001
☏(0471) 2478397. Fax : 91-471-2473496

**B. JAIN PUBLISHERS (P) LTD.
INDIA**

> **NOTE FROM THE PUBLISHERS**
> Any information given in this book is not intended to be taken as a replacement for medical advice. Any person with a condition requiring medical attention should consult a qualified practitioner or therapist.

PREVENTIVE & SOCIAL MEDICINE

© All rights are reserved

No part of this publication may be reproduced, stored in a retrieval system or transmitted, in any form or by any means, mechanical, photocopying, recording or otherwise, without prior written permission of the publishers.

First Edition : 2002

Price: Rs. 110.00

Published by

Kuldeep Jain

for

B. Jain Publishers (P) Ltd.

1921, Chuna Mandi, St. 10th Paharganj,
New Delhi-110 055
Ph: 3670430, 3670572, 3683200, 3683300
Fax: 011-3610471 & 3683400
Website: www.bjainbooks.com, Email: bjain@vsnl.com

PRINTED IN INDIA

by

Unisons Techno Financial Consultants (P) Ltd.
522, FIE, Patpar Ganj, Delhi-110 092

ISBN : 81-7021-1116-X
BOOK CODE : B-5563

CONTENTS

II B.H.M.S. 1993 1

II B.H.M.S. 1994 37

II B.H.M.S. 1995 63

II B.H.M.S. 1996 89

II B.H.M.S. 1997 129

II B.H.M.S. 1998 167

II B.H.M.S. 1999 185

II B.H.M.S. 2000 217

II B.H.M.S. 2001 247

II B.H.M.S. 1993

PART A

Q.1. Describe the natural history of disease in man.

Ans. Natural history of disease: The term natural history of disease signifies the way in which a disease evolves over time from the earliest stage of its prepathogenesis phase to its termination as recovery, disability or death in the absence of treatment or prevention.

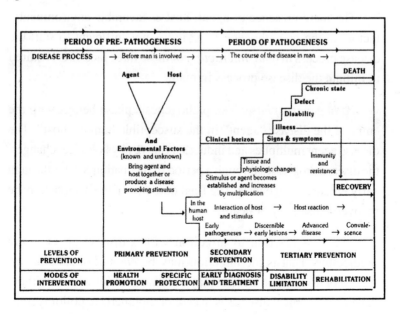

The natural history of disease consists of two phases:—

1. Prepathogenesis phase.
2. Pathogenesis phase.

Prepathogenesis phase: This refers to the period preliminary to the onset of disease in man. The disease agent has not yet entered man; but the factors which favor its interaction with the human host are already existing in the environment.

The causative factors of disease may be classified as:—

(i) Agent.
(ii) Host.
(iii) Environment.

These three factors are referred to as the *epidemiclogical triad.*

The mere presence of agent, host & favorable environmental factors in the prepathogenesis period is not sufficient to start the disease process in man. *Interaction* of these three factors is required to initiate the disease process in man.

Pathogenesis phase: The pathogenesis phase beings with the entry of the disease "agent" in the susceptible human "host". The disease agent multiplies and induces tissue & physiological changes, the disease progresses through a period of incubation & later through early & late pathogenesis. The final outcome of the disease may be recovery, disability or death.

The host reaction to infection with a disease agent is not predictable. That is the infection may be *clinical* or *subclinical; typical* or *atypical* or the host may become a carrier with or without developing clinical disease as in case of diphtheria & poliomyelitis.

In chronic diseases (e.g., coronary heart disease, hypertension, cancer), the early pathogenesis phase is less dramatic. This phase in chronic disease is referred to as the presymptomatic phase. During this presymptomatic phase there is no manifest disease. The pathological changes are below "clinical horizon". The clinical stage begins when recognizable signs & symptoms appear.

Levels of prevention:—
1. Primary prevention
2. Secondary prevention.
3. Tertiary prevention.

Primary prevention: It can be defined as action taken prior to the onset of disease, which removes the possibility that disease will ever occur. It signifies the intervention in the prepathogenesis phase or a disease or health problem.

Primary prevention may be accomplished by measures designed to promote general health, well-being & quality of life in people or by specific protective measures.

The WHO has recommended the following approaches for primary prevention of chronic diseases:—

(a) Premordial prevention: Prevention of the emergence or development of risk factors in countries or population groups in which they have not yet appealed. For e.g., smoking, eating patterns.

(b) Population (mass) Strategy: It is directed at the whole population irrespective of individual risk factors. For e.g., studies have shown that even a small reduction in the average blood pressure of a population would produce a large reduction in cardiovascular diseases.

(c) High-risk strategy: It aims to bring preventive care to individuals at special risk. This requires detection of individuals at high risk by optimum use of clinical methods.

Secondary prevention: "Action which halts the progress of a disease at its incipient stage & prevents complications".

The specific interventions are:—

(a) Early diagnosis (e.g., screening tests, case finding programmes).
(b) Adequate treatment.

By early diagnosis and adequate treatment, secondary prevention attempts to arrest the disease process, restore health by seeking out unrecognized disease and treating it before reversible pathological changes have taken place.

3. *Tertiary prevention:* It signifies intervention in the late pathogenesis phase. Tertiary prevention can be defined as all measures available to reduce or limit impairments and disabilities. For e.g., treatment even if undertaken late in the natural history of a disease may prevent the sequelae and limit disability.

Modes of intervention:—

(i) Health Promotion.
(ii) Specific Protection.
(iii) Early diagnosis and treatment.
(iv) Disability limitation.
(v) Rehabilitation.

(i) *Health promotion:* It is the process of enabling people to increase control over and to improve health. It is not directed against any particular disease, but is intended to strengthen the host through a variety of approaches (interventions). The well known interventions in this area are:—

(a) Health education.
(b) Environmental modifications.
(c) Nutritional interventions.
(d) Lifestyle and behavioral changes.

(a) Health education: A large number of diseases could be prevented if people are adequately informed about them and if they are encouraged to take necessary precautions in time.

(b) Environmental modifications: Such as provision of safe water; installation of sanitary latrines; control of insects and rodents; improvement of housing, etc.

(c) Nutritional interventions: These comprise of food distribution and nutritional improvement of vulnerable groups, child feeding programmes, food fortifications, nutritional education, etc.

(d) Lifestyle and behavioral changes: The action of prevention in this case is one of individual and community responsibility for health. The physician and each health worker acts as an educator, rather than a therapist.

(ii) *Specific protection:* To avoid disease altogether is the ideal 2but this is possible only in a limited number of cases. The following are some of the currently available interventions aimed at specific protection:—

(a) Immunization.
(b) Use of specific nutrients.
(c) Chemoprophylaxis.
(d) Protection against occupational diseases.
(e) Protection against accidents.
(f) Protection against carcinogens.
(g) Avoidance of allergens.
(h) The control of specific hazards in general environment.

(iii) *Early diagnosis and treatment:* Are main interventions of disease control. The earlier a disease is diagnosed and treated the better it is from the point of view of prognosis and preventing the occurrence of further cases or any longterm disability.

(iv) *Disability limitation:* When a patient reports late in the pathogenesis phase the mode of intervention is disability limitation.

Concept of disability:—

Disease

↓

Impairment

↓

Disability

↓

Handicap

Impairment: Any loss or abnormality of psychological, physiological or anatomical structure or functions.

E.g., loss of foot, defective vision.

Disability: Because of an impairment, the affected person may be unable to carry out certain activities considered normal for his age, sex, etc.

Handicap: It is defined as a disadvantage for a given individual, resulting from an impairment or a disability that limits or prevents the fulfillment of a role that is normal.

(v) *Rehabilitation:* Defined as the combined and coordinated use of medical, social, educational and vocational measures for training and retraining the individual to the highest possible level of functional ability.

Q.2 How will you carry out a nutritional survey in a slum colony of Delhi? Discuss the various methods to assess health status of under-five children?

Ans. Nutritional survey: In nutritional surveys the examination of a random and representative sample of the population covering all ages and both sex in different socio-economic groups is sufficient to be able to draw valid conclusions.

Assessment methods:—

1. Clinical examination.
2. Anthropometry.
3. Biochemical evaluation.
4. Functional assessment.

5. Assessment of dietary intake.
6. Vital and health statistics.
7. Ecological studies.

1. *Clinical examination:* It is an essential feature of all nutritional surveys since their ultimate objective is to assess levels of health of individuals or of population groups in relation to food they consume. There are a number of physical signs, some specific and many non-specific, known to be associated with states of malnutrition. However clinical signs have the following drawbacks:—

(a) Malnutrition cannot be quantified on the basis of clinical signs.
(b) Many deficiencies are unaccompanied by physical signs.
(c) Lack of specificity and subjective nature of most of the physical signs.

2. *Anthropometry:* Anthropometric measurements such as height, weight, skin fold thickness and arm circumference are valuable indications of nutritional status. If anthropometric measurements are recorded over a period of time, they reflect the patterns of growth and development and how individuals deviate from the average at various ages in body size, build and nutritional status.

3. *Biochemical assessment:—*

(a) Laboratory tests:—
    (i) Hb estimation: It is an important laboratory test that is carried out in nutritional surveys.

(ii) Stool and urine: Stool should be examined for intestinal parasites. Urine should examined for albumin and sugar.

(b) Biochemical tests: With increasing knowledge of the metabolic functions of vitamins and minerals, assessment of nutritional status by clinical signs has given way to more precise biochemical tests.

Some biochemical tests in nutritional surveys are:—

Nutrient	Method	Normal value
Vit. A	Serum retinol	20 mcg/dl
Thiamine	Thiamine pyrophosphate (TPP) stimulation of RBC transketolase activity.	1.00-1.23 (ratio)
Riboflavin	RBC glutathione reductase activity stimulated by FAD	1.0-1.2 (ratio)
Niacin	Urine N-methyl nicotinamide	(not reliable)
	Serum folate	6.0 mcg/ml
	Red cell folate	160 mcg/ml
Vit. B_{12}	Serum Vit. B_{12} concentration	160 mg/l
Vit. C	Leucocyte ascorbic acid	15 mcg/10^8 cells
Vit. K	Prothrombin time	11-16 seconds

Biochemical tests are expensive and time consuming so they are usually applied in a sub-population.

4. *Functional indicators:* Functional indices of nutritional status are emerging as an important class of diagnostic tools. Some of the functional indicators are given in the table below:—

System	Nutrients
1. Structural integrity	
Erythrocyte fragility	Vit. E, Se
Capillary fragility	Vit. C
Tensile strength	Cu
2. Host defense	
Leucocyte chemotaxis	P/E, Zn
Leucocyte phagocytic capacity	P/E, Fe
Leucocyte bactericidal capacity	P/E, Fe, Se
T cell blastogenesis	P/E, Zn
Delayed cutaneous hypersensitivity	P/E, Zn
3. Hemostasis	
Prothrombin time	Vit. K
4. Reproduction	
Sperm count	Energy, Zn
5. Nerve function	
Nerve conduction	P/E, Vit. B, Vit. B_{12}
Dark adaptation	Vit. A, Zn
EEG	P/E
6. Work capacity	
Heart rate	P/E, Fe
Vasopressor response	Vit. C

5. *Assessment of dietary intake:—*

A dietary survey may be carried out by one of the following methods:—

(i) Weighing of raw foods: The survey team visits the house-hold and weighs all food that is going to be cooked and eaten as well as that which is wasted or discarded. The duration may vary from 1 to 2! days but commonly 7 days which is called one dietary cycle.

(ii) Weighing of cooked food.

(iii) Oral questionaire method: Inquiries are made retrospectively about the nature and quantity of foods eaten during the previous 24 to 48 hours.

The data collected has to be transformed into:—

(a) Mean intake of food in terms are cereals, pulses, vegetables, fruits, milk, meat, fish and eggs.

(b) The mean intake of nutrients per adult man value or consumption unit.

6. *Vital statistics:* An analysis of vital statistics – mortality and morbidity data – will identify groups at high risk and indicate the extent of risk to community.

7. *Assessment of ecological factors:* A study of ecological factors comprises the following:—

(i) Food balance sheets: In this supplies are related to census population to derive levels of food consumption in terms of per capita supply availability.

(b) Socio-economic factors: Are like family size, occupation, income, education, customs, cultural patterns in relation to feeding practices of children.

(c) Health and educational services: PHC services, feeding and immunization programmes should also be taken into consideration.

(d) Conditioning influences: These include parasitic, bacterial and viral infections which precipitate malnutrition.

Health status of under-five children can be assessed by the following methods:—

1. *Weight:* Infants born to well-fed mothers in India weigh about 3.2 kg at birth.

   Baby doubles its birth weight by 5 months of age, trebles it by 1 year. By the end of 2nd year birth weight gets quadrupled.

2. *Height:* In first year of life, the body lengths by about 50%. In the second year another 12 to 13 cms are added. After that growth is 5-6 cms every year.

3. *Head and chest circumference:* At birth, the head circumference is larger than the chest circumference.

4. *Growth chart:* It is the visible display of the child's physical growth and development, child should be weighed atleast once every month during the first year.

Every 2 month during second year, and every 3 month thereafter till 5 to 6 years of age. When the child's weight is plotted on the growth chart at monthly intervals against his or her age, it gives *weight-for-age* growth curve.

Q.3 Describe the heath problems associated with high socioeconomic status. Discuss preventive and control measures for these diseases.

Ans. Health problems associated with high socio-economic status are:—

(a) CHD.

(b) Hypertension.

(c) Cancer.

(d) Diabetes mephitis.

(e) Obesity.

(a) *CHD:* Personality which is prone to CHD is mesomorphic, aggressive, hard driving, restless with staccato speech. He is competitive.

Predisposing risk factors for CHD are:—

1. Hypertension.
2. Heavy smoking.
3. Diabetes mellitus.
4. Mental stress.
5. Obesity.
6. Excessive intake of saturated fats, cholesterol and alcohol.
7. Thyrotoxicosis.
8. Sedentary habits, lack of regular exercise and irregular ways of life.
9. Gout.

Preventive and control measures:—

1. Population strategy or primary prevention.
   (i) Prevention in whole population.
   (ii) Primordial prevention.
2. High risk strategy.
3. Secondary prevention.

1. Population strategy or primary prevention:—
(i) Prevention in whole population: Include following specific interventions:—
(a) Dietary changes:—
- Reduction of fat intake to 20-30%.
- Consumption of saturated fatty acid must be limited to less than 10% of total energy intake.
- A reduction of dietary cholesterol to below 100 mg per 1000 Kcal per day.
- An increase in complex carbohydrate consumption.
- Avoidance of alcohol consumption; reduction of salt intake to 5g daily or less.

(b) Smoking: The goal is to achieve a smokeless society.
(c) B.P.: Even a small reduction in the average B.P. of the whole population by a mere 2 to 3 mm Hg would produce a large reduction in the incidence of cardiovascular complications.
(d) Physical activity: Regular physical activity should be a part of normal daily life.
(ii) Premordial prevention: It involves preventing the emergence

and spread of CHD risk factors and lifestyles that have not yet appeared or become endemic.

2. High risk strategy:—

(i) Identifying the risk: By simple tests such as B.P. and serum cholesterol measurements.

(ii) Specific advice: The next step is to bring them under preventive care and motivate them into taking a positive action against all the identified risk factors.

3. Secondary prevention: Are like drug trials, coronary surgery, use of pace makers and all the preventive measures discussed above.

(b) *Hypertension:* May be primary (essential) whose exact etiology is not known or secondary in which factors for hypertension are renal, adrenal gland tumors, toxemias of pregnancy, etc.

Predisposing factors:—

1. Hereditary and familial tendency.
2. Obesity.
3. Stress and strains in life.
4. Worry and nervous tension.
5. Overeating esp. saturated fats and high salt intake.
6. Alcohol smoking, tobacco chewing.

Prevention and control measures:—

1. There must be a routine B.P. record of every patient.
2. Heavy smoking and excessive alcohol drinking should be avoided.

3. One should learn to live with unavoidable worry, tension and strain in life.
4. Proper diet control.
5. All these factors should be stressed on the public through health education, primary health centers.

(c) *Cancer:* The etiology of cancer is not known exactly.

Contributory agent factors:—

1. Chemical agents
   - Organic – Coal tar, aniline dyes, etc.
   - Inorganic – Asbestos, nickel, etc.

2. Physical agents eg., X-ray, ultra violet rays and radiations.

3. Nutritional agents eg., polyunsaturated fats when kept for long as such or after heating are oxidized and tend to develop mutagenic and carcinogenic substances.

4. Mechanical agents eg., friction, trauma, etc.

Contributory factors in man:—

1. Age: Incidence of cancer is more with advance in age although some cancers like leukemia occur in young as well.
2. Sex: Lung and esophageal cancer → males.
   Breast cancer → females.
3. Some cancers are associated with the occupation.
4. Hereditary and environmental factors.

Prevention and control:—

1. Try to avoid and protect against known carcinogenic agents.

2. Ensure proper personal hygiene.
3. Health education.
4. Early cancer detection. People should also have awareness about salient features which need detection and investigation. These are: chronic swelling, lump in breast, hoarseness, excessive menstrual bleeding.
5. Persons in old age should be encouraged and motivated for regular medical checkups

(d) *Diabetes mellitus:* Clinical diabetes is manifested by hyperglycemia and glycosuria due to deficient or lack of insulin secretion or its ineffectiveness which results in impaired metabolism of the nutrients.

Prevention and control:—

1. Detection of prediabetic cases, which show impaired glucose tolerance curve.
2. Diet control.
3. Maintenance of standard weight.
4. Known diabetics should be motivated for proper treatment and maintenance.
5. Proper health education.

(e) *Obesity:* Common causes are:—

Overeating and sedentary habits.

Prevention:—

1. No overeating.
2. Regular daily exercise.

3. Avoid saturated fats, sugar.
4. No eating between the meals.
5. No alcohol.
6. Dietary therapy preferred to so called drug therapy.

PART B

Q.4 Discuss the health hazards of ingestion/ chewing/ smoking of tobacco.

Ans. Tobacco chewing and tobacco smoking causes:—

1. Oral cancer.
2. Lung cancer.
3. Coronary heart disease.
4. Hypertension.

1. Oral cancer: Occur among those who smoked or chewed tobacco. Oral cancer is preceded by some type of precancerous lesion. Cancer almost always occurred on the side of mouth where tobacco quid was kept. Precancerous stage precedes the development of cancer.

2. Lung Cancer: Tobacco smoking is the main cause of lung cancer. There is a relationship between cigarette smoking and lung cancer. *The risk is strongly related to:—*

(a) The number of cigarettes smoked.
(b) The age of starting to smoke.
(c) Smoking habits.

(d) Puffs, the nicotine and tar content.

(e) Length of cigarettes.

Those who are highly exposed to "passive smoking" are at increased risk of developing lung cancer. The most noxious component of tobacco smoke are tar, carbon monoxide and nicotine. The carcinogenic agent is tar. Nicotine and CO, particularly contribute to increased risk.

3. *Coronary heart disease:* Are associated with smoking tobacco because it contains carbon monoxide which induces atherogenesis; nicotine stimulates the adrenergic drive raising both B.P. and myocardial oxygen demand; lipid metabolism with fall in "protective" high-density lipoproteins, etc.

4. *Hypertension:* Smoking, chewing tobacco may contribute to hypertension.

Q.5 Describe the life cycle of lice and name the disease caused by lice infection in man. Describe its prevention.

Ans. Life cycle of lice:—

1. Eggs.
2. Larva.
3. Adult

Eggs: Are laid singly or in groups, firmly attached to the hair or lining of clothing by a cementing substance. The eggs are small, ovoid bodies, pointing at one end and truncated and pitted at the other end. Eggs hatch in 6 to 9 days.

Larva: Looks very much like an adult except smaller in size. Larval stage may take 10 to 15 days.

Adult: The entire life cycle from an egg to adult takes 10-15 days.

The diseases caused by lice infection are:—

(i) Epidemic typhus.

(ii) Relapsing fever.

(iii) Trench fever.

(iv) Dermatitis.

Prevention:—

1. Improvement in personal hygiene.
2. A daily bath with soap and water is essential to prevent lice.
3. Woman with long hair should wash and clean their hair frequently.
4. Clothing, towels and sheets should be washed with hot water.

Q.6 What sanitary measures will you take for the Kumbh mela with an expected attendance of 50 lakh population?

Ans. Sanitary measures are:—

1. *Before the mela:—*

(a) Selection of site: The health officer and district engineer should go to the fair site for selection of site and preparation of the necessary programme for lodging houses, proper conservancy, water supply, general sanitation and the required equipment. Roads should be marked and repaired.

(b) General arrangement: All necessary materials like brooms, strings, lime and bleaching powder should be stored in godowns.

(c) Staff required and materials:—

    (i) Medical officer – one.

    (ii) Health inspector – one.

    (iii) One sweeper for every 1000 people for trench latrine.

    (iv) One sweeper for every 5000 person per day for picking up from the road.

    (v) One sweeper for every 2000 person per day for collecting rubbish and dumping it.

    (vi) Some extra sweepers dealing with other urgent matters.

    (vii) Disinfectants.

(d) Water supply: Adequate and safe water supply is of utmost important.

(e) Refuse and conservancy system: Bore hole latrines are very suitable and hygienic for the purpose. It must reach 1 feet below the sub-soil water. Dustbins, urinals and soakage pits etc. should be provided at suitable places.

2. *During the mela:—*

(a) Water Supply: Wells should be regularly disinfected. If water has been found unfit for drinking, it should be made undrinkable by pouring kerosene oil on them, or keeping a watch so that nobody drinks that unfit water. Water should be drawn by special men with proper buckets. Inspecting staff should have test tubes, potassium iodide crystals and starch powder to test the presence of chlorine and to know whether the wells have been disinfected properly or not.

(b) Refuse disposal: The refuse and road sweepings should be disposed off properly.

(c) Conservancy: Male and female latrines should be marked. They should be lighted during the night. Sweepers should be posted at each latrine for cleaning and filling the used latrine. Bleaching powder and lime should be sprinkled freely. People should be prevented from passing stool on the ground.

(d) Food sanitation: The sale of stale food, unripe and over-ripe fruits should not be permitted. One medical officer should be authorized to seize any unwholesome articles of food and destroy the same.

(e) Accommodation: There should not be over-crowding in rooms; sick people should be moved to the hospital.

(f) Medical care: Dispensaries should be under a competent medical officer. Arrangement for emergencies should be made.

PART C

Q.7 Discuss the tuberculosis control programme. Describe its preventive measures.

Ans. The National Tuberculosis Programme: It has been in operation since 1962. The goal of NTP is to reduce the problem of tuberculosis in the community sufficiently quickly to the level where it ceases to be a public health problem.

District Tuberculosis Programme (DTP) is the backbone of NTP. The District Tuberculosis Centre (DTC) is the nucleus to DTP. The function of the DTC is to plan, organize and implement the DTP in the entire district in association with general health services.

Their activities include:—

(a) *Case finding:* Sputum examination is done to detect new T.B. cases in rural population. To further improve case finding male health workers are required to collect and fix sputum of the symptomatic cases on the slide during their routine visits to the villages and send the slides to the nearest health center for microscopic examination.

(b) *Treatment:* It is free and is offered on domiciliary basis from all the health institutions. It is organized in such a manner that patients are expected to collect drugs once a month on fixed dates from the nearest treatment centre. When the patient fails to collect his/her drugs on the "due date", a letter is written to him/her and in the event of no response for 7 days a home visit is paid by the hospital staff.

(c) *BCG vaccination:* By UIP, the coverage of BCG has gone up.

(d) *Recording and reporting:* The names and addresses of all the sputum the cases are sent to DTC every Saturday. The DTC registers all sputum positive cases.

(e) *Supervision:* The DTC team visits the peripheral health institutions regularly and helps them in planning and rendering T.B. control services.

The DTC team includes:—

1 District tuberculosis officer.

1 Laboratory technician.

1 Treatment organiser.

1 X-ray technician.

1 Non-medical team leader.

1 Statistical assistant.

Prevention and control of T. B.:—

1. It should be a compulsorily notifiable disease.
2. All the sputum positive patients should be isolated till they are sputum negative.
3. All detected cases should be promptly treated with a proper follow up to ensure the continuity of their treatment.
4. Chemoprophylaxis of all known contacts should be undertaken.
5. Early diagnosis and detection of cases.
6. Rehabilitation of the treated cases.
7. Health education of the public so that they should endeavour to avoid exposure to infection and cooperate in BCG vaccination and chemoprophylaxis, etc.
8. Some of the practical methods under the mass screening programme are as follows:—

(i) Mass tuberculin testing is useful in establishing index of infection in a given community.

(ii) Sputum examination for AFB. This is one of the easiest and fruitful methods to uncover many undetected tubercular cases.

(iii) BCG vaccination should be given to new borns below four weeks and the other susceptible individuals to protect against the infection.

Q.8 (a) Describe the cold chain in the National Immunization Programme at a health centre.

(b) Write short notes on:—

(i) IMR.
(ii) MMR.
(iii) Nutritional deficiency anemia.
(iv) Hypervitaminosis.
(v) Sex education at school age.
(vi) Mid-day meal programme.

Ans. (a) Cold chain: The cold chain is a system of storage and transport of vaccines at low temperature from the manufacturer to the actual vaccination site. The cold chain system is necessary because vaccine failure may occur due to a failure in storing and transporting the vaccine under strict temperature controls. The cold chain equipment consist of:—

(i) Cold box: It is meant to transport large quantities of vaccine by vehicle to out of reach sites.
(ii) Vaccine carrier: It is meant to transport small quantities of vaccine by bicycle or by foot.
(iii) Flasks: They are used if vaccine carriers are not available.
(iv) Ice-packs.
(v) Refrigerator.

(b) (i) IMR: It is defined as the ratio of infant death registered in a given year to the total number of live births registered in the same year, usually expressed as a rate per 1000 live births.

$$\text{IMR} = \frac{\text{Number of deaths of children less than 1 year of age in a year}}{\text{Number of live births in same year}} \times 1000$$

Factors contributing to infant mortality:—

1. Biological factors:—

(a) Birth weight: A satisfactory birth weight is required for infant survival.

(b) Age of mother: Under 20 years and over 30 years mothers are at greater risk to cause infant mortality.

(c) Order of birth: Highest mortality is found among first births. The fate of the 5th child worse than the 3rd.

(d) Interval between births: The shorter the time interval between birth, greater the risk to survival of the infant.

(e) Multiple births: Infants born in multiple births face a greater risk of death.

2. Economic factors:—

Low socio-economic people have high IMR.

3. Cultural and social factors:—

(a) Breast feeding reduces IMR.

(b) Illiteracy increase IMR.

(c) Sex of child: A female child is unwelcome in the family.

(d) Broken families have high IMR.

(e) Lack of trained personals.

Prevention:—

1. Prenatal feeding: Improve the physical well being of the pregnant women.
2. Immunization: Of mother and child is very important.
3. Growth monitoring.
4. Breast feeding.
5. Family planning.
6. Efficient MCH services.
7. Improvement in the standard of living.

(ii) MMR: It is defined as death of a woman when pregnant or within 42 days of termination of pregnancy, irrespective of the duration and site of pregnancy from any cause related or aggravated by pregnancy.

$$MMR = \frac{\text{Total number of female deaths due to complications of pregnancy, child birth or within 42 days if delivery from puerperal causes in an area during a given year}}{\text{Total no. of live birth in same year.}} \times 1000$$

Causes:—

1. Toxemias of pregnancy.
2. Hemorrhage.
3. Infection.
4. Induced abortion.
5. Obstructed labor.
6. Anemia.

7. Other related diseases eg., cardiac, renal, etc.

Prevention:—

1. Dietary supplementation.
2. Prevention of infection and hemorrhage.
3. Prevention of complications eg., eclampsia, malpresentations.
4. Treatment of medical conditions eg., hypertension.
5. Promotion of family planning.
6. Anti-malaria and tetanus prophylaxis.

(iii) Nutritional deficiency anemia: It is a disease syndrome caused by malnutrition in its widest sense. A condition in which Hb. content of blood is lower than normal as a result of a deficiency of one or more essential nutrients, regardless of the cause of such deficiency.

Iron deficiency can arise either due to an inadequate intake or poor bioavailability of dietary iron or due to excessive losses of iron from the body.

Interventions:—

An estimation of Hb should be done to assess the degree of anemia.

If anemia is "severe", high doses of iron or blood transfusion may be necessary. The other interventions are:—

Iron and folic acid supplementation. In order to prevent anemia, Govt. of India has launched the National Nutritional Anemia Prophylaxis Programme during the fourth five year plan. The programme is based on daily supplementation with iron and folic acid tablets to prevent mild and moderate cases of anemia.

The iron and folic acid tablets are given to high risk groups like pregnant mothers, lactating mothers, children below 12 years.

Dosage:—

Mothers: One tablet of iron and folic acid containing 60 mg of elemental iron and 0.5 mg of folic acid. The daily administration should be continued until 2 to 3 months.

Children: Screening test for anemia may be done on infants at 6 months, and 1 and 2 years of age. One tablet of iron and folic acid containing 20 mg of elemental iron and 0.1 mg of folic acid should be given daily.

(iv) Hypervitaminosis: An excess intake of vitamin than the required and storing capacity causes hypervitaminosis. An excess intake of ratinol causes nausea, vomiting, anorexia and sleep disorders followed by skin desquamation and then an enlarged liver and papillary edema. High intakes of carotene may color plasma and skin but do not appear to be dangerous since vitamin A can be stored in the body for 6 to 9 months and liberated slowly, its excess can cause hypervitaminosis. Vitamin D is stored in the body in fatty tissues and in the liver. An excessive intake is harmful and may result in anemia, nausea, vomiting, thirst and drowsiness. The patient may lapse into coma, while cardiac arrhythmias and renal failure may occur. The effects are due to hypercalcemia induced by increased intestinal absorption and mobilization of calcium from bone.

(v) Sex education at school age: Children should be given sex education at school age by their teachers and their course should also include the sex education because of so many sexually transmitted diseases like AIDS, Syphilis, etc., Due to lack of knowledge, the students are curious towards sex and they want to experiment with it. This way they ruin there life by causing harm to their health and their careers and by the time they realize their mistakes, it is too late. Later they are guilty conscious. To prevent children from the hazards of lack of knowledge, the teachers should give them sex education so that they get familiar with it and no curiosity is left in them. They should also be taught about STD.

(vi) Mid-day meal programme: It is in operation since 1961 throughout the country. The major objective of the programme is to attract more children for admission to schools and to retain them so that literacy improvement children could be brought about. The following broad principle should be kept in mind:—

(a) The meals should be a supplement and not a substitute to the home diet.

(b) The meal should supply at least one-third of the total energy requirement and half of the protein needed.

(c) The cost of the meal should be reasonably low.

(d) The meal should be such that it can be prepared easily in schools.

(e) As far as possible, locally available foods should be used.

(f) The menu should be changed frequently to avoid monotony.

Q.9 (a) Describe the etiology, pathology, prevention and complications of measles.

(b) Write short notes on:—

(i) Differences between health center and dispensary.

(ii) Control of nutritional deficiency diseases in antenatal clinic.

(iii) Milestones of a child upto 5 years.

(iv) Prevention of nutritional blindness.

(v) Fly control measures.

Ans. (a) Etiology:—

Causative organism: Virus belong to the myxovirus group, present in nasopharyngeal secretions and in blood of infected persons.

Source of infection: Nasopharyngeal secretions of the patients. No carriers.

Mode of spread:—
(i) Droplet infection.
(ii) Through fomites.

Pathology:—

Diseases is more prevalent in children.

Clinical features:—

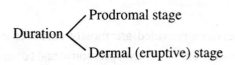

Prodromal period lasts from 2-5 days, during which there is a sudden onset of fever with catarrhal symptoms.

Diagnostic lesions during this period are the *Koplick's spots* which appear on the buccal mucous membrane in the form of whitish spots surrounded by a reddish base.

Dromal (eruptive) stage begins by the 4th or 5th day when a maculo-papular rash appears on the face, trunk and extremities. This gradually fades by the 6th or 7th day.

Complications:—

(i) Bronchopneumonia.

(ii) Encephalitis.

(iii) Gastroenteritis.

(iv) Otitis media.

Prevention:—

Isolation of the patients and quarantine of the contacts.

The use of measles vaccination for active immunization and of immunoglobulins for prevention of infection in susceptible children. Measles vaccine is given around 9 months-1 year for effective prevention.

(b) (i) Differences between in health centre and dispensary: A Dispensary differs from a health centre in the following respects:—

(a) In a dispensary, services provided are mostly curative; in a health center the services are preventive, promotive and curative, all integrated.

(b) A dispensary has no catchment area i.e. it has no definite area of responsibility. Patients may be drawn from any part of the country. A health centre on the other hand, is responsible for a definite area and population.

(c) The health team in a health centre is a optimum "mix" of medical and paramedical workers; in a dispensary the team consists of only the curative staff i.e. doctors, compounders, nurses, etc.

(ii) Control of nutritional deficiency diseases in antenatal clinic: The main nutritional deficiency diseases in antenatal clinic are:—

Anemia: The major etiological factors being iron and folic acid deficiencies, causing high incidence of premature births, postpartum hemorrhage, puerperal sepsis and thromboembolic phenomena in mother.

The Government of India has initiated a programme in which 60 mg of elemental iron and 500 mcg of folic acid are being distributed daily to pregnant mothers.

Protein and vitamin deficiency: To control this fresh milk or skimmed milk is provided to pregnant mothers free of cost. Capsules of Vitamin A and D are also supplied.

(iii) Milestones of a child upto 5 years:—

MILESTONES OF DEVELOPMENT

	Motor Development	Language development	Adaptive development	Socio-personal development
6-8 weeks				Looks at mother & smiles.
3 months	Holds head erect.			
4-5 months		Listening.	Begins to reach out for objects.	Recognizes mother.
6-8 months	Sits without support.	Experimenting with noise.	Transfers objects hand to hand.	Enjoys hide and seek.
9-10 months	Crawling.	Increasing range of sounds.	Releases objects.	Suspicious of strangers.
10-11 months	Stands with support.	First words.		

12-14 months	Walks with wide base.		Builds.
18-21 months	Walks with narrow base; beginning to run.	Joining words together.	Beginning to explore.
2 years	Runs.	Short sentences	Day by day.

Ideally children should be weighed at least once every month during the first year; every 2 months during the second year and every 3 months thereafter upto 5 to 6 years. The weight should be plotted on a growth chart against his or her age, as it gives weight for age curve.

(iv) Prevention of nutritional blindness: Malnutrition due to vitamin A deficiency can result in permanent blindness.

To prevent nutritional blindness:—

(a) Vitamin A prophylaxis programme: National Programme for Control of Blindness is to administer a single massive dose of an oily preparation of Vitamin A containing 200,000 IU orally to all preschool children in the community every 6 months.

(b) Fortification of foods with Vitamin A like Dalda, sugar, etc.

(c) Health education to people for primary eye care.

(d) Persuading people in general and mothers in particular, to consume generally green leafy vegetables and other Vitamin A rich foods.

(e) Promotion of breast feeding.

(v) Fly control measures:—

(a) *Environmental control:—*

(i) Storing garbage, kitchen wastes and other refuse in bins with tight lids.

(ii) Efficient collection, removal and disposal of refuse by incineration, compositing and sanitary land fill.

(iii) Provision of sanitary latrines.

(iv) Stopping open-air defecation.

(v) Sanitary disposal of animal excreta.

(b) *Insecticidal control:—*

(i) Residual sprays: DDT, lindane, fenthion, malathion. The addition of sugar to insecticidal formulations enhances their effectiveness.

(ii) Baits: Poisoned baits contain 1 or 2 percent diazinon; malathion, liquid baits contain 0.1 to 0.2%; same for insecticides and 10% sugar water. The cheapest bail is one that is made by mixing 3 teaspoons of formalin with one pint of H_2O.

(iii) Cords and ribbons: Impregnated with diazinon, fenthion have been tried with success.

(iv) Space sprays: They contain pyrethrin, DDT or HCH.

(c) *Fly papers:—*

It is made by mixing of zibs resin and one point of castor oil. It is heated until the mixture resembles molasses. This is smeared on paper by using an ordinary paint brush.

(d) *Protection against flies:* Screening of houses, hosptitals, food markets, etc. Screens with meshes to the inch will keep out houseflies.

(e) *Health education.*

II B.H.M.S. 1994

PART A

Q.1 Describe in detail all levels of prevention in relation to any chronic disease of national importance in India.

Ans. Levels of prevention:—

1. Primary prevention
2. Secondary prevention.
3. Tertiary prevention.

Primary prevention: It can be defined as action taken prior to the onset of disease, which removes the possibility that disease will ever occur. It signifies the intervention in the prepathogenesis phase or a disease or health problem.

Primary prevention may be accomplished by measures designed to promote general health, well-being & quality of life in people or by specific protective measures.

The WHO has recommended the following approaches for primary prevention of chronic diseases:—

(a) Premordial prevention: Prevention of the emergence or development of risk factors in countries or population groups in which they have not yet appealed. For e.g., smoking, eating patterns.

(b) Population (mass) Strategy: It is directed at the whole population irrespective of individual risk factors. For e.g., studies have shown that even a small reduction in the average blood pressure of a population would produce a large reduction in cardiovascular diseases.

(c) High-risk strategy: It aims to bring preventive care to individuals at special risk. This requires detection of individuals at high risk by optimum use of clinical methods.

Secondary prevention: "Action which halts the progress of a disease at its incipient stage & prevents complications".

The specific interventions are:—

(a) Early diagnosis (e.g., screening tests, case finding programmes).
(b) Adequate treatment.

By early diagnosis and adequate treatment, secondary prevention attempts to arrest the disease process, restore health by seeking out unrecognized disease and treating it before reversible pathological changes have taken place.

3. *Tertiary Prevention:* It signifies intervention in the late pathogenesis phase. Tertiary prevention can be defined as all measures available to reduce or limit impairments and disabilities. For e.g., treatment even if undertaken late in the natural history of a disease may prevent the sequelae and limit disability.

A chronic disease of national importance in India is Tuberculosis:—

Primary prevention:—

(a) Premordial prevention: Discouraging the emergence or development of risk factors in the country like air pollution, crowding of houses, smoking, eating roadside food, etc.

(b) Population strategy: Changing the lifestyles like development of socio-economic status, health education about T.B., regular checkups, vaccination (BCG) to the children under EPI.

(c) High risk strategy: Preventive care to individuals at risk like doctors, detection of high risk groups by clinical methods, contacts of T.B. cases, nurses, etc.

Secondary prevention:—

Early diagnosis and treatment by screening tests and case finding programmes.

Case finding is done by:—

(i) Sputum examination by primary health centre workers.

(ii) Tuberculin test.

Treatment is by chemotherapy. The objective of treatment is elimination of both fast and slowly multiplying bacilli.

Tertiary prevention: It is done to limit the damage to the lungs or other organs due to T.B.

Q.2 Discuss the quality of food from sanitation and hygiene aspects in respect to food served in:—

   (a) Five star hotels;

   (b) Dhabas;

   (c) Halwai shops;

   (d) Households.

Ans. (a) Five star hotels: If the hotel is situated away from filth, open drains, stable, manure pits, etc. it is very good according to sanitation and hygiene aspect. The food which is cooked in hotels is not fresh but it is not reached by flies. Ventilation is there in the rooms. Rooms are very clean. However food sanitation also depend on personal hygiene and habits of food handlers. The handlers should wash their hand every time they serve. Also the sanctation and hygiene of utensils in which food is served is improtant.

(b) Dhabas: These are usually situated near some open drain. There is no ventilation. The utensils are not clean. The food handlers are not cleanly dressed. Flies suround the food and the rooms are not very clean. A dhaba is usually very congested. Hence, the food served in dhaba is not good according to sanitation and hygiene.

(c) Halwai shops: These are always reached by flies. These flies contaminate the food. Rats live in these shops and contaminate the food. Food is not fresh. Rooms are not clean. There is no ventilation. The utensils are not clean. Food handlers are not educated and they don't know anything about personal hygiene. So food served in a halwai shop is also bad according to sanitation and hygiene.

(d) Households: At home, food is good according to sanitation and hygiene because fresh vegetables which are washed properly are used. The food is never touched by flies. Home is a clean place to eat the food. The personal hygiene maintained is very good for sanitation of food, utensils are also cleaned properly. So, the food which we cook ourself and eat in our home is best according to hygiene and sanitation.

Q.3 Discuss the following:—

(a) Protein calorie malnutrition.

(b) Criterion for selection of a prize baby in a baby show.

Ans. (a) Protein calorie malnutrition: It is a major health problem in India. It occurs particularly in weaklings and children in the first years of life. It is not only an important cause of childhood mortality and morbidity, but also leads to permanent impairment of physical and possibly of mental growth.

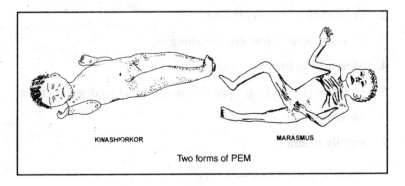

Two forms of PEM

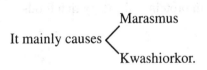

Causes:—

(a) Inadequate intake of food, both in quantity and quality.
(b) Infections notably diarrhea, respiratory infections, measles, intestinal worms.
(c) Poor environmental conditions.
(d) Large family.
(e) Poor maternal health.
(f) Failure of lactation.
(g) Premature termination of breast feeding.

The first indication of PCM is *being underweight for age.*

Preventive measures are:—

Health promotion:—

1. Measures directed to pregnant and lactating mothers.
2. Promotion of breast feeding.
3. Development of low-cost weaning foods.
4. Measures to improve family diet.
5. Nutritional education – promotion of correct feeding practices.
6. Health economics.
7. Family planning.

Specific protections:—

1. Child's diet must contain protein and energy rich foods.
2. Immunization.
3. Food fortification.

Early diagnosis and treatment:—

1. Periodic surveillance.
2. Early diagnosis of lag in growth.
3. Early diagnosis and treatment of infections and diarrhea.
4. Development of programmes for early rehydration of children with diarrhea.

Rehabilitation:—
1. Nutritional rehabilitation services.
2. Hospital treatment.
3. Follow up care.

(b) Criteria for selection of a prize baby in a baby show, where you are a medical officer on its selection board:—

In a good baby show for selection of a prize baby there are the following things:—

(i) Registration: All infants and babies are to be registered.
(ii) Medical examination: Complete medical examination including height and weight are measured. The child is examined for evidence of disease or defects.
(iii) Parent counseling: About the diet, sleep, test, habits, etc.
(iv) Immunization: Child must be immunized against the six dreadful diseases.
(v) Activeness of the child.
(vi) His vision and hearing capacity, walking, etc.

PART B

Q.4 Discuss in detail various methods used for chlorination of water. What measures will you take in an epidemic of gastroenteritis in a town?

Ans. Chlorination of water: Chlorination is one of the greatest advances in water purification. Various methods of chlorination are:—

(1) *Chlorine gas:* It is cheap, quick in action, efficient and easy to apply. It is applied by a special equipment called chlorinating equipment. It is the method of first choice.

(2) *Chloramines:* These are loose compounds of chlorine and ammonia. They have a less tendency to produce chlorinous taste and give a more persistent type of residual chlorine. The greatest drawbacks of chloramines is that they have a slower action than chlorine so it is not used to a great extent in water treatment.

(3) *Perchloran:* It is a calcium compound which carries 60-70% of available chlorine.

The following measures will be employed to check gastroenteritis epidemic:—

(1) *Notification:* Early notification is very important. An outbreak of gastroenteritis should be notified immediately by telegram to the district health authority, state and national health authority.

(2) *Isolation of the case:* In the hospital or in the house should be done. The contacts should be segregated and treated.

(3) *Sterilization of water:* The water supplies should be protected from contamination and immediate disinfection of those supplies which are believed to be exposed to risk of pollution. The water may be sterilized by:—

(i) Chlorination

(ii) Permanganate of potash.

(iii) Boiling.

(4) *Protection of food:* Food should be well cooked and properly protected from flies, dust, etc. Uncooked food should be avoided and no one should be allowed to handle food without thoroughly washing and disinfecting their hands.

(5) *Fly control:* By DDT, malathion spray.

(6) *Disposal of night soil:* Indiscrete defecations should be avoided or stopped. Quick and effective disposal of night soil should be done, so that flies may not come in contact with night soil.

(7) *Disinfection:* Concurrent and terminal disinfection is required. Bleaching powder can be used.

(a) Stools and vomit: All excreta and vomit should be collected in a basin and mixed with an equal quantity of 5% cresol or 3% bleaching powder. After two hours of disinfection it should be burnt or buried.

(b) Clothings and beddings: The cloth should be soaked in 2½% cresol solution for ½ an hour and then washed with soap and water.

(c) Floors and walls: The floor must be thoroughly disinfected with

5% cresol. The walls upto a height of 3 feet should be treated similarly.

(d) Cooking utensils: Disinfected by boiling for 15 minutes or keeping them in cresol solution for ½ hour before washing finally with water and soda.

(e) Hands: Dipped in 1% cresol.

8. *Vaccination.*

9. *Health education.*

Q.5 How will you sterilize or disinfect the following:—

(a) Cotton in your clinic.
(b) Clinical thermometer after use by a leprosy patient.
(c) Gloves after delivery of an AIDS patient.
(d) Instruments after a gyne checkup of a patient having venereal disease.
(e) Sputum of a T. B. patient.
(f) Telephone used by a diphtheria patient.
(h) Ornaments exposed to an AIDS infection.
(h) Leather jacket.

Ans (a) Cotton in your clinic: Cotton can disposed of by:—

(i) Incineration or burning.
(ii) Dumping.
(iii) Controlled tipping.

Incineration is the most common method. The cotton refuse is collected in dustbins.

(b) **Clinical thermometers after use by a leprosy patient:** The thermometer is sterilized by autoclaving.

(c) **Gloves after delivery of an AIDS patient:** Autoclaving and boiling for 5-10 minutes above 90 degrees is suitable to sterilize the gloves.

(d) **Instruments after a gynae checkup of a patient having venereal disease:—**
   (i) Autoclaving.
   (ii) Boiling.

(e) **Sputum of a T.B. patient:** It is received in a gauze or paper handkerchief and destroyed by burning.

If the amount is considerable it is disinfected by boiling or autoclaving for 20 minutes.

(f) **Telephone used by a diphtheria patient:** It is disinfected by formaldehyde gas.

(g) **Ornaments exposed to an AIDS infection:** These ornaments are sterilized by autoclaving.

(h) **Leather jacket:—**
   (i) Boiling.
   (ii) Autoclaving.

Q.6 Describe the methods for control of mosquitoes.

Ans. Mosquito Control Measures:—

1. *Anti-larval measures:—*

(a) Environmental control: Reducing their breeding places. This is known as source reduction and comprises of minor engineering methods such as filling, leveling and drainage of breeding places:—

Culex: Reducing domestic and predomestic sources of breeding such as cesspools and open ditches.

Aedes: Environment should be cleaned up and got rid of water holding containers such as discarded tins, empty pots, broken bottles, etc.

Anopheles: Breeding places should be looked for and abolished by appropriate engineering measures.

Mansonia: Reduce the aquatic plants.

(b) Chemical control: Commonly used larvicides are:—

   (i) Mineral oils.

   (ii) Paris green.

   (iii) Synthetic insecticides.

Mineral oils: The application of oil to water is one of the oldest known mosquito control measures. Since the life cycle of a mosquito occupies about 8 days or so it is customary to apply oil once a week on all breeding places.

Paris green: It is a stomach poison and to be effective it must be ingested by the larvae. Anopheles are surface feeders so it is easily killed by Paris green and for bottom feeders Paris green is applied in granular formation.

Synthetic insecticides: E.g., fenthion, chlorpyrifos and abate are effective larvicides. These organophosphorus compounds hydrolyze quickly in water.

(c) Biological control: A wide range of small fish feed readily on mosquito larvae. The best known are Gambusia offense and Lebister reticulatus.

2. *Anti-adult measures:—*

(a) Residual sprays: E.g., DDT 1-2 grams of pure DDT per sq. metre are applied 3 times a year to walls and other surfaces where mosquitoes rest.

(b) Space sprays: These are those where the insecticidal formulation is sprayed into the atmosphere in the form of mist or fog to kill insects.

Common space sprays are:—

(i) Pyrethrum extract: Pyrethrum flowers form an excellent space sprays.

It has the active principle *pyrethrin* which is a nerve poison and kills the insects instantly on mere contact.

(ii) Residual insecticide: Malathion and jenitrothin.

(c) Genetic control:—

   (i) Sterile male technique.

   (ii) Cytoplasmic incompatibility.

   (iii) Chromosomal translocations.

   (iv) Sex distortion.

   (v) Gene replacement.

3. *Protection against mosquito bites:—*

(a) Mosquito net: It offers protection against mosquito bites during sleep. The net should be white to allow easy detection of mosquitoes. Best pattern is a rectangular net.

The size of opening should not exceed 0.0475 inch in diameter. The number of holes in one square inch are usually 150.

(b) **Screening:** Of buildings with copper or bronze gauze having 16 meshes to the inch is recommended. The aperture should not be larger than 0.0475 inch.

(c) **Repellents:** Like Diethyl toluamide is active against fatigans.

PART C

Q.7 Discuss the role of a homoeopathic doctor in the control of:—

(a) Malaria.

(b) Leprosy.

(c) AIDS.

(d) Rabies.

Ans. (a) Malaria: A homoeopathic physician should educate his patients about the various precautions to be taken in order to prevent malaria. Maintaining proper hygiene, not letting the water to stand, keeping the water coolers clean, sleeping in mosquito nets, using effective reppelants, etc., are some of the precautions.

When a patient of suspected malaria comes to a homoeopathic physician he should investigate the case by getting the various blood studies done including peripheral smear for malarial parasite.

When malaria is confirmed, the doctor should start the appropriate remedies.

(b) Leprosy: The role of homoeopathic physician are as follows:—

(i) The doctor should detect the case of leprosy among his patients as early as possible.
(ii) If the case is positive then he should refer the patient to a good hospital which specializes in leprosy treatment.
(iii) Also the patient should be educated for proper compliance.
(iv) The public should be made aware that leprosy is curable and it is not a hereditory diseases.

(c) AIDS: A suspected case of HIV should be first sent for a sensitive test. Then a confirmatory test is done in form of *Western Blot* which is a ELISA test. Proper education should be imparted regarding awarding indiscriminate sex, using condom. One should not share razors and toothbrushes. IV users should not share needles and syringes.

(d) Rabies: The patient should be isolated in quite room protected from external stimuli. The patient should be made comfortable to relieve his anxiety. Appropriate remedies should be started.

Q.8 What will you advice to an antenatal woman in your clinic? Describe the diet of a pregnant woman.

Ans. A major component of antenatal care is antenatal advice:—

(i) *Diet:* Pregnancy in total duration consumes about 60,000 Kcal, over and above the normal metabolic requirements. On an average 12 kg weight gain occurs during pregnancy. So, the pregnant woman should take a balanced and adequate diet.

(ii) *Personal hygiene:*—

    (a) Personal cleanliness: She should bathe every day and wear clean clothes.

    (b) Rest and sleep: 8 hours sleep and at least 2 hours rest after a mid day meal.

    (c) Bowels: Constipation should be avoided by regular intake of green leafy vegetables.

    (d) Exercise: Light exercise.

    (e) No smoking.

    (f) Maintain oral hygiene.

    (g) Sexual intercourse restricted during pregnancy.

(iii) *Drugs:* She should not take any drugs without consulting the doctor.

(iv) *Radiation:* No X-rays should be done during pregnancy.

(v) *Warning signs:* Mother should be given clear-cut instructions that she should immediately report when:—

    (a) Swelling of feet.

    (b) Fits.

    (c) Headache.

    (d) Blurring of vision.

    (e) Bleeding per vagina.

    (f) Any other unusual symptoms.

(vi) *Child care:* Advice on hygiene and child rearing.

(vii) *Family planning.*

(viii) *Immunization against tetanus.*

Diet of a pregnant woman:—

The pregnancy diet should be light, nutritious, easily digestible and rich in protein, minerals and vitamins. The diet should consist of principal food along with one litre of milk, one egg, plenty of green vegetables and fruits available. At least, half of the total protein should be first class and majority of fat should be animal type. Supplementary iron therapy is needed for all pregnant mothers. One tablet daily of ferrous sulphate containing 60 mg of elemental iron is recommended.

Recommended daily nutrients for a pregnant woman:—

Kilocalories	2500
Protein	60 g
Calcium	1000 mg
Iron	40 mg
Vitamin A	6000 IU
Vitamin D	400 IU
Thiamine	1.5 mg
Riboflavine	1.5 mg
Nicotinic acid	15 mg
Ascorbic acid	60 mg

Folic acid 1 mg

Vitamin B_{12} 2µg

Q.9 Describe in brief:—

(a) Crude birth rate.

(b) Maternal mortality rate.

(c) Safe sex.

(d) B.C.G.

(e) Primary health center.

(f) Filaria control.

Ans. (a) Crude birth rate: It is defined as the number of birth per 1000 mid year population per year in a given community.

$$\text{Birth rate} = \frac{\text{Number of live births during the year}}{\text{estimated mid year population}} \times 1000$$

The birth rate is an unsatisfactory measure of fertility because the total population is not exposed to child bearing.

(b) Maternal mortality rate (MMR): It is defined as death of a woman when pregnant or within 42 days of termination of pregnancy, irrespective of the duration and site of pregnancy from any cause related or aggravated by pregnancy.

$$\text{MMR} = \frac{\text{Total number of female deaths due to complications of pregnancy, child birth or within 42 days if delivery from puerperal causes in an area during a given year}}{\text{Total no. of live birth in same year}} \times 1000$$

Causes:—

1. Toxemias of pregnancy.
2. Hemorrhage.
3. Infection.
4. Induced abortion.
5. Obstructed labor.
6. Anemia.
7. Other related diseases eg., cardiac, renal, etc.

Prevention:—

1. Dietary supplementation.
2. Prevention of infection and hemorrhage.
3. Prevention of complications eg., eclampsia, malpresentations.
4. Treatment of medical conditions eg., hypertension.
5. Promotion of family planning.
6. Anti-malaria and tetanus prophylaxis.

(c) **Safe sex:** It is defined as the use of contraceptive measures at the time of sex to avoid unwanted births and to control the time at which births occur in relation to the age of parents. These also provide some protection against sexually transmitted diseases, a reduction in the incidence of pelvic inflammatory diseases and possibly some protection from the risk of cervical cancer. The best method for safe sex is use of the condom. It is the widely known and used barrier device by the males around the world. It is marked by Govt. as Nirodh in India.

For females, *intrauterine device* are best for safe sex. These include *copper devices* like Copper T; only follow up care is needed.

The ideal IUD candidate:—

(i) Who has borne atleast one child.

(ii) Has no history of pelvic disease.

(iii) Has normal menstrual history.

(iv). Is willing to check IUD tail.

(v) Has access to follow up and treatment of potential problems.

(vi) Is in a monogamous relationship.

(d) B.C.G: This is the vaccination given to infants to fight against tuberculosis.

It is given at the time of birth. BCG must be protected from exposure to light during storage.

Dosage: For vaccination the usual strength is 0.1 mg in 0.1 ml volume.

Administration: The standard procedure recommended by WHO is to inject the vaccine intradermally using a *"Tuberculin"* syringe.

Age: BCG is administer at the time of birth.

Phenomena after vaccination: Two or three weeks after a correct intradermal injection of a potent vaccine, a papule develops at the site of vaccination. It increases slowly in size upto 4 to 8 mm in 5 weeks. It then subsides or breaks into a shallow ulcer, rarely open but usually seen covered with a crust. Healing occurs spontaneously within 6 to 12 weeks leaving a permanent, tiny scar.

Complications:—

(a) Prolonged severe ulceration at the site of vaccination.

(b) Suppurative lymphadenitis.

(c) Osteomyelitis.

(d) Disseminated BCG infection.

(e) Death.

Protective value: Duration of protection is 15-20 years.

(e) Primary health center:—

The Bhore committee in 1946 gave the concept of primary health center as a basic health unit, to provide, as close to the people as possible, an integrated curative and preventive health care to rural population with emphasis on preventive and promotive aspects of health care.

One PHC for every 30,000 rural populations in the plains and one PHC for every 20,000 population in hilly, tribal and backward area.

Function of PHC:—

(i) Medical care.

(ii) MCH including family planning.

(iii) Safe water and basic sanitation.

(iv) Prevention and control of locally endemic diseases.

(v) Collection and reporting of vital statistics.

(vi) Education about health.

(vii) National health Programmes.

(viii) Referral services.

(ix) Training of health guides, health workers, local dais and health assistants.

(x) Basic laboratory services.

Staffing pattern at PHC level:—

Medical officer	1
Pharmacist	1
Nurses/midwife	1
Health worker (female)	1
Block extension educator	1
Health assistant (male)	1
Health assistant (female)	1
UDC	1
LDC	1
Lab technician	1

Driver	1
Class IV	4
Total	**15**

(f) Filaria control:—

The prevention is based on:—

(a) Chemotherapy.

(b) Vector control.

Chemotherapy: Action of drugs against microfilariae and the adult worms in human host.

Vector control: Mosquito Control Measures.

1. *Anti-larval measures:—*

(a) Environmental control: Reducing their breeding places. This is known as source reduction and comprises of minor engineering methods such as filling, leveling and drainage of breeding places:—

Culex: Reducing domestic and predomestic sources of breeding such as cesspools and open ditches.

Aedes: Environment should be cleaned up and got rid of water holding containers such as discarded tins, empty pots, broken bottles, etc.

Anopheles: Breeding places should be looked for and abolished by appropriate engineering measures.

Mansonia: Reduce the aquatic plants.

(b) Chemical control: Commonly used larvicides are:—

   (i) Mineral oils.

   (ii) Paris green.

   (iii) Synthetic insecticides.

Mineral oils: The application of oil to water is one of the oldest known mosquito control measures. Since the life cycle of a mosquito occupies about 8 days or so it is customary to apply oil once a week on all breeding places.

Paris green: It is a stomach poison and to be effective it must be ingested by the larvae. Anopheles are surface feeders so it is easily killed by Paris green and for bottom feeders Paris green is applied in granular formation.

Synthetic insecticides: E.g., fenthion, chlorpyrifos and abate are effective larvicides. These organophosphorus compounds hydrolyze quickly in water.

(c) Biological control: A wide range of small fish feed readily on mosquito larvae. The best known are Gambusia offense and Lebister reticulatus.

2. *Anti-adult measures:*—

(a) Residual sprays: E.g., DDT 1-2 grams of pure DDT per sq. metre are applied 3 times a year to walls and other surfaces where mosquitoes rest.

(b) Space sprays: These are those where the insecticidal

formulation is sprayed into the atmosphere in the form of mist or fog to kill insects.

Common space sprays are:—

(i) Pyrethrum extract: Pyrethrum flowers form an excellent space sprays.

It has the active principle *pyrethrin* which is a nerve poison and kills the insects instantly on mere contact.

(ii) Residual insecticide: Malathion and jenitrothin.

(c) Genetic control:—

   (i) Sterile male technique.

   (ii) Cytoplasmic incompatibility.

   (iii) Chromosomal translocations.

   (iv) Sex distortion.

   (v) Gene replacement.

3. *Protection against mosquito bites:—*

(a) Mosquito net: It offers protection against mosquito bites during sleep. The net should be white to allow easy detection of mosquitoes. Best pattern is a rectangular net.

The size of opening should not exceed 0.0475 inch in diameter. The number of holes in one square inch are usually 150.

(b) Screening: Of buildings with copper or bronze gauze having 16 meshes to the inch is recommended. The aperture should not be larger than 0.0475 inch.

(c) Repellents: Like Diethyl toluamide is active against fatigans.

II B.H.M.S. 1995

PART A

Q.1 Discuss the role of social and cultural factors in disease and health.

Ans. Social factors: Many diseases are common in low socio-economic groups because of:—

1. Poverty.
2. Insufficient education.
3. Lack of knowledge regarding the nutritive value of foods, inadequate sanitary environment, large family size, etc.

Diseases related to high socio-economic group are:—

1. Obesity, which is due to over-nutrition and overeating.
2. Hypertension.
3. CHD.
4. Diabetes.

Disease related to low socio-economic group are:—

1. Malnutrition: It is largely the by product of poverty, lack of

knowledge, etc. These factors bear most directly on the quality of life.

2. Rheumatic heart disease.
3. Tuberculosis.
4. Intestinal parasites.

Social factors also have an influence on human health. Health status is determined primarily by the level of socio-economic development.

Those of major importance are:—

(i) *Economic status:* The per capita GNP is the most widely accepted measure of general economic performance. It is the economic progress that has been the major factor in reducing morbidity, increasing life expectancy and improving the quality of life.

The economic status determines the purchasing power, standard of living, quality of life, family size, pattern of disease and deviant behavior in the community. It is also an important factor in seeking health care.

(ii) *Education:* A second major factor influencing health status is education. The world map of illiteracy closely coincides with maps of poverty, malnutrition, ill health, high infant and child mortality rates.

(iii) *Occupation:* The very state of being employed in productive works promotes health because the unemployed usually show a higher incidence of ill health and death.

(iv) *Political system:* Health is also related to the country's political system.

Cultural Factors:—

(a) *Food habits, customs, beliefs, traditions and attitudes:* Food habits are the oldest and most deeply entrenched aspects of any culture. They have deep psychological roots and are associated with love, affection and warmth. The family plays an important role in shaping habits and their habits are passed from one generation to the other.

Rice is a stable cereal in eastern and southern states. The crux of the problem is that many customs and beliefs apply most often to vulnerable groups i.e. infants, toddlers, expectant and lactating women.

(b) *Religion:* It has a powerful influence on the food habits of the people. Hindus do not eat beef and Muslims pork. Some orthodox Hindus and Jains do not eat meat, fish, eggs and onion. These are known as food taboos which prevent people from consuming nutritious foods even when these are available easily.

(c) *Food fads:* In the selection of food, personal likes and dislikes also play a major role.

(d) *Cooking practices:* Draining away the rice water at the end of cooking, prolonged boiling in open pans influence the nutritive value of food.

Q.2 How will you assess the nutritional status of a community?

Ans. In nutritional surveys the examination of a random and representative sample of the population covering all ages and both sex in different socio-economic groups is sufficient to be able to draw valid conclusions.

Assessment methods:—
1. Clinical examination.
2. Anthropometry.
3. Biochemical evaluation.
4. Functional assessment.
5. Assessment of dietary intake.
6. Vital and health statistics.
7. Ecological studies.

1. *Clinical examination:* It is an essential feature of all nutritional surveys since their ultimate objective is to assess levels of health of individuals or of population groups in relation to food they consume. There are a number of physical signs, some specific and many non-specific, known to be associated with states of malnutrition. However clinical signs have the following drawbacks:—

(a) Malnutrition cannot be quantified on the basis of clinical signs.
(b) Many deficiencies are unaccompanied by physical signs.
(c) Lack of specificity and subjective nature of most of the physical signs.

2. *Anthropometry:* Anthropometric measurements such as height, weight, skin fold thickness and arm circumference are valuable indications of nutritional status. If anthropometric measurements are recorded over a period of time, they reflect the patterns of growth and development and how individuals deviate from the average at various ages in body size, build and nutritional status.

3. **Biochemical assessment:—**

(a) Laboratory tests:—

  (i) Hb estimation: It is an important laboratory test that is carried out in nutritional surveys.

  (ii) Stool and urine: Stool should be examined for intestinal parasites. Urine should examined for albumin and sugar.

(b) Biochemical tests: With increasing knowledge of the metabolic functions of vitamins and minerals, assessment of nutritional status by clinical signs has given way to more precise biochemical tests.

Some biochemical tests in nutritional surveys.

Nutrient	Method	Normal value
Vit. A	Serum retinol	20 mcg/dl
Thiamine	Thiamine pyrophosphate (TPP) stimulation of RBC transketolase activity.	1.00-1.23 (ratio)
Riboflavin	RBC glutathione reductase activity stimulated by FAD	1.0-1.2 (ratio)
Niacin	Urine N-methyl nicotinamide	(not reliable)
	Serum folate	6.0 mcg/ml
	Red cell folate	160 mcg/ml
Vit. B_{12}	Serum Vit. B_{12} concentration	160 mg/l
Vit. C	Leucocyte ascorbic acid	15 mcg/10^8 cells
Vit. K	Prothrombin time	11-16 seconds

Biochemical tests are expensive and time consuming so they are usually applied in a sub-population.

4. *Functional indicators:* Functional indices of nutritional status are emerging as an important class of diagnostic tools. Some of the functional indicators are given in the table below:—

System	Nutrients
1. Structural integrity	
Erythrocyte fragility	Vit. E, Se
Capillary fragility	Vit. C
Tensile strength	Cu
2. Host defense	
Leucocyte chemotaxis	P/E, Zn
Leucocyte phagocytic capacity	P/E, Fe
Leucocyte bactericidal capacity	P/E, Fe, Se
T cell blastogenesis	P/E, Zn
Delayed cutaneous hypersensitivity	P/E, Zn
3. Hemostasis	
Prothrombin time	Vit. K
4. Reproduction	
Sperm count	Energy, Zn
5. Nerve function	
Nerve conduction	P/E, Vit. B, Vit. B_{12}
Dark adaptation	Vit. A, Zn
EEG	P/E
6. Work capacity	
Heart rate	P/E, Fe
Vasopressor response	Vit. C

5. *Assessment of dietary intake*:—

A dietary survey may be carried out by one of the following methods:—

(i) Weighing of raw foods: The survey team visits the house-hold and weighs all food that is going to be cooked and eaten as well as that which is wasted or discarded. The duration may vary from 1 to 21 days but commonly 7 days which is called one dietary cycle.

(ii) Weighing of cooked food.

(iii) Oral question aire method: Inquiries are made retrospectively about the nature and quantity of foods eaten during the previous 24 to 48 hours.

The data collected has to be transformed into:—

(a) Mean intake of food in terms are cereals, pulses, vegetables, fruits, milk, meat, fish and eggs.

(b) The mean intake of nutrients per adult man value or consumption unit.

6. *Vital statistics:* An analysis of vital statistics – mortality and morbidity data – will identify groups at high risk and indicate the extent of risk to community.

7. *Assessment of ecological factors:* A study of ecological factors comprises the following:—

(i) Food balance sheets: In this supplies are related to census population to derive levels of food consumption in terms of per capita supply availability.

(b) Socio-economic factors: Are like family size, occupation, income, education, customs, cultural patterns in relation to feeding practices of children.

(c) Health and educational services: PHC services, feeding and immunization programmes should also taken into consideration.

(d) Conditioning influences: These include parasitic, bacterial and viral infections which precipitate malnutrition.

Health status of under-five children can be assessed by the following methods:—

1. *Weight:* Infants born to well-fed mothers in India weigh about 3.2 kg at birth.

   Baby doubles its birth weight by 5 months of age, trebles it by 1 year. By the end of 2nd year birth weight gets quadrupled.

2. *Height:* In first year of life, the body lengths by about 50%. In the second year another 12 to 13 cms are added. After that growth is 5-6 cms every year.

3. *Head and chest circumference:* At birth, the head circumference is larger than the chest circumference.

4. *Growth chart:* It is the visible display of the child's physical growth and development, child should be weighed atleast once every month during the first year.

   Every 2 month during second year, and every 3 month thereafter till 5 to 6 years of age. When the child's weight is plotted on the growth chart at monthly intervals against his or her age, it gives *weight-for-age* growth curve.

Q.3 Name the milk borne diseases. Describe the methods of pasteurization of milk.

Ans. Milk borne diseases are:—

(1) *Infections of animals that can be transmitted to man:—*

(a) Tuberculosis.
(b) Brucellosis.
(c) Streptococcal infections.
(d) Staphylococcal enterotoxin poisoning.
(e) Salmonellosis.
(f) Q fever.
(g) Cowpox.
(h) Foot and mouth disease.
(i) Anthrax.
(j) Leptospirosis.
(k) Tick borne encephalitis.

(2) *Infections primary to man that can be transmitted through milk:—*

(a) Typhoid.
(b) Shigellosis.
(c) Cholera.
(d) Enteropathogenic Escherichia Coli (EEC).

Methods of pasteurization:—

(1) *Holder method:* In this process, milk is kept at 63-66° C for at least 30 minutes and then quickly cooled to 5° C. It is recommended for small communities.

(2) *HTST method:* "High temperature and short time method". Milk is rapidly heated to a temperature nearly 72° C and is hold at that temperature for not less than 15 seconds and rapidly cooled to 4° C.

(3) *UHT method:* Ultra high temperature method. Milk is rapidly heated in usually 2 stages (the second stage usually being under pressure) to between 125° C for a few seconds only. It is then rapidly cooled and bottled as quickly as possible.

PART B

Q.4 Describe a water filteration plant.

Ans. Rapid sand or mechanical filters: The following steps are involved in the purification of water by rapid sand filters:—

(1) *Coagulation:* Raw water is treated with coagulants such as alum; the dose varies from 5-40 milligrams or more per litre depending upon the turbidity and color, temperature and the pH value of the water.

(2) *Rapid mixing:* The treated water is then subjected to violent agitation in a "mixing chamber" for a few minutes. This allows a quick and thorough dissemination of alum throughout the bulk of water which is very necessary.

(3) *Flocculation:* The next phase involves a slow and gentle stirring of the treated water in a "flocculation chamber" for about 30 minutes. The mechanical flocculator consists of a number of paddles which rotate at 2 to 4 spins rotate with the help of motors. This slow and gentle stirring results in the formation of thick copious white flocculant precipitate of aluminium hydroxide.

(4) *Sedimentation:* The coagulated water is now led into the sedimentation tanks where it is detained for periods varying from 2-6 hours. At least 95% of the flocculent precipitate needs to be removed before the water is admitted into rapid sand filters. The sludge which settles at the bottom and is removed from time to time.

(5) *Filtration:* The clarified water is now subjected to rapid sand filtration.

Filter beds: Each unit of filter bed has a surface of about 80 to 90 m^2 Sand is the filtering medium; effective size of sand particles is between 0.6-2.0 mm.

Depth of sand bed is about 1 metre. Below the sand bed is a layer of graded gravel 30 to 40 cm deep.

As filtration proceeds, the "alum floc" not removed by sedimentation is held back on the sand bed. It forms a slimy layer. It adsorbs bacteria from the water and effects purification. Oxidation of ammonia also takes place during passage of water through the filters. As filtration proceeds the suspended impurities and bacteria clog the filters. The filters soon become dirty and begin to loose their efficiency.

(6) *Back washing:* It is done daily or weekly. Reversing the flow

of water through the sand bed is called back-washing. It disposes the impurities and cleans up the sand bed.

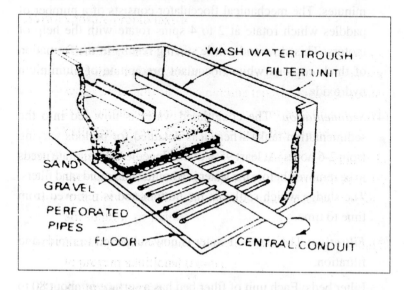

Q.5 Name the various types of non-service latrines. Which type will you recommended for rural areas? Describe it in detail.

Ans. Non-service type:—

(a) Bore hole latrine.

(b) Dug well or pit latrine.

(c) Water seal type of latrines.

    (i) P.R.A.I. type.

    (ii) R.C.A. type.

    (iii) Sulabh shauchalya.

(d) Septic tank.

(e) Aqua privy.

We will recommend the water seal type latrine in rural areas.

Essential features of R.C.A. latrine are described below:—

(1) *Location:* It should not be located within 15 m from a source of water supply, it should be at a lower elevation to prevent bacterial contamination of water supply.

(2) *Squatting plate:* It should be made of impervious material so that it can be washed and kept completely dry.

(3) *Pan:* Retrieves night soil urine and wash water. The length of pan is 17 inches. The width of the front portion of the pan is minimum 5 inches and width at its widest part is 8 inches.

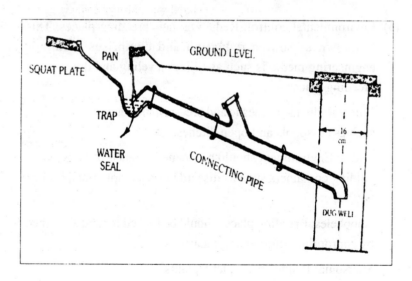

(4) *Trap:* It is a bent pipe about 7.5 cm in diameter and is connected with the pan. It holds the water and provides necessary "water seal". It is a distance between the level of water in the trap and

the lowest point in the concave upper surface of the trap. Water seal is 2 cm and it prevents the access by flies and suppresses the nuisance from smell.

(5) *Connecting pipes:* When the pit is dug away from the squatting plate so connecting pipes are required to join them.

(6) *Dug well:* Or pit is usually deep and is covered.

(7) *Superstructure:* It is used to provide privacy.

Q.6 Discuss the role of various insecticides in the National Malaria Control Programme.

Ans. Mosquito Control Measures:—

1. *Anti-larval measures:—*

(a) Environmental control: Reducing their breeding places. This is known as source reduction and comprises of minor engineering methods such as filling, leveling and drainage of breeding places;—

Culex: Reducing domestic and predomestic sources of breeding such as cesspools and open ditches.

Aedes: Environment should be cleaned up and got rid of water holding containers such as discarded tins, empty pots, broken bottles, etc.

Anopheles: Breeding places should be looked for and abolished by appropriate engineering measures.

Mansonia: Reduce the aquatic plants.

(b) Chemical control: Commonly used larvicides are:—

   (i) Mineral oils.

   (ii) Paris green.

(iii) Synthetic insecticides.

Mineral oils: The application of oil to water is one of the oldest known mosquito control measures. Since the life cycle of a mosquito occupies about 8 days or so it is customary to apply oil once a week on all breeding places.

Paris green: It is a stomach poison and to be effective it must be ingested by the larvae. Anopheles are surface feeders so it is easily killed by Paris green and for bottom feeders Paris green is applied in granular formation.

Synthetic insecticides: E.g., fenthion, chlorpyrifos and abate are effective larvicides. These organophosphorus compounds hydrolyze quickly in water.

(c) Biological control: A wide range of small fish feed readily on mosquito larvae. The best known are Gambusia offense and Lebister reticulatus.

2. *Anti-adult measures:*—

(a) Residual sprays: E.g., DDT 1-2 grams of pure DDT per sq. metre are applied 3 times a year to walls and other surfaces where mosquitoes rest.

(b) Space sprays: These are those where the insecticidal formulation is sprayed into the atmosphere in the form of mist or fog to kill insects.

Common space sprays are:—

(i) Pyrethrum extract: Pyrethrum flowers form an excellent space sprays.

It has the active principle *pyrethrin* which is a nerve poison and kills the insects instantly on mere contact.

(ii) Residual insecticide: Malathion and jenitrothin.

(c) Genetic control:—
- (i) Sterile male technique.
- (ii) Cytoplasmic incompatibility.
- (iii) Chromosomal translocations.
- (iv) Sex distortion.
- (v) Gene replacement.

3. *Protection against mosquito bites:—*

(a) Mosquito net: It offers protection against mosquito bites during sleep. The net should be white to allow easy detection of mosquitoes. Best pattern is a rectangular net.

The size of opening should not exceed 0.0475 inch in diameter. The number of holes in one square inch are usually 150.

(b) Screening: Of buildings with copper or bronze gauze having 16 meshes to the inch is recommended. The aperture should not be larger than 0.0475 inch.

(c) Repellents: Like Diethyl toluamide is active against fatigans.

PART C

Q.7 Describe the National Tuberculosis Control Programme.

Ans. The National Tuberculosis Programme: It has been in operation since 1962. The goal of NTP is to reduce the problem of tuberculosis in the community sufficiently quickly to the level where it ceases to be a public health problem.

District Tuberculosis Programme (DTP) is the backbone of NTP. The District Tuberculosis Centre (DTC) is the nucleus to DTP. The function of the DTC is to plan, organize and implement the DTP in the entire district in association with general health services.

Their activities include:—

(a) *Case finding:* Sputum examination is done to detect new T.B. cases in rural population. To further improve case finding male health workers are required to collect and fix sputum of the symptomatic cases on the slide during their routine visits to the villages and send the slides to the nearest health center for microscopic examination.

(b) *Treatment:* It is free and is offered on domiciliary basis from all the health institutions. It is organized in such a manner that patients are expected to collect drugs once a month on fixed dates from the nearest treatment centre. When the patient fails to collect his/her drugs on the "due date", a letter is written to him/her and in the event of no response for 7 days a home visit is paid by the hospital staff.

(c) *BCG vaccination:* By UIP, the coverage of BCG has gone up.

(d) *Recording and reporting:* The names and addresses of all the sputum the cases are sent to DTC every Saturday. The DTC registers all sputum positive cases.

(e) *Supervision:* The DTC team visits the peripheral health institutions regularly and helps them in planning and rendering T.B. control services.

The DTC team includes:—

1 District tuberculosis officer.

1 Laboratory technician.

1 Treatment organiser.

1 X-ray technician

1 Non-medical team leader.

1 Statistical assistant.

Prevention and control of T. B.:—

1. It should be a compulsorily notifiable disease.
2. All the sputum positive patients should be isolated till they are sputum negative.
3. All detected cases should be promptly treated with a proper follow up to ensure the continuity of their treatment.
4. Chemoprophylaxis of all known contacts should be undertaken.
5. Early diagnosis and detection of cases.
6. Rehabilitation of the treated cases.
7. Health education of the public so that they should endeavour to avoid exposure to infection and cooperate in BCG vaccination and chemoprophylaxis, etc.
8. Some of the practical methods under the mass screening programme are as follows:—

(i) Mass tuberculin testing is useful in establishing index of infection in a given community.

(ii) Sputum examination for AFB. This is one of the easiest and fruitful methods to uncover many undetected tubercular cases.

(iii) BCG vaccination should be given to new borns below four weeks and the other susceptible individuals to protect against the infection.

Q.8 Name the diseases transmitted by indiscriminate defecation. Describe prevention and control of any one of them.

Ans. Diseases transmitted by indiscriminate defection are:—

(a) Typhoid fever.

(b) Paratyphoid fever.

(c) Dysenteries.

(d) Diarrhea.

(e) Cholera.

(g) Hookworms.

(h) Ascariasis.

(i) Infective hepatitis.

(j) Prevention and control of hookworm

Prevention and control involves four approaches:—

1. Sanitary disposal of feces.
2. Chemotherapy.
3. Correction of anemia.

4. Health education.

1. *Sanitary technology*: Long term solution of the problem is the sanitary disposal of human excreta through the installation of sewage disposal system in urban areas. This alone will prevent soil pollution.

2. *Chemotherapy*: Periodic case finding and treatment of all infected persons in the community will reduce the worm burden and frequency of transmission.

3. *Treatment of anemia*: When anemia is severe it should be treated. A cheap and effective treatment is ferrous sulphate 200 mg, three time a day, orally and continued upto 3 months after the Hb has risen to 12 g/100ml.

4. *Health education:* Community involvement through health education is an important aspect in the control of hookworm infection. Health education should be aimed at the use of sanitary latrines and prevention of soil pollution.

Q.9 Write short notes on:—

(i) AIDS.

(ii) Under-five clinic.

(iii) Copper T.

Ans. (i) AIDS:—

Causative organism: Human Immunodeficiency Virus (HIV)

Incubation period: 6 months to 10 years.

Mode of spread:—

(a) Virus is transmitted through blood and other body fluids.

(b) Anal intercourse.

(c) Habitual intravenous drug users.

(d) Prostitutes.

(e) Pregnant mother suffering from this disease pass it on to the babies.

Course of disease:—

(1) Initial infection: Some patients have symptoms of fluor glandular fever, others have no symptoms upto a few years. However, infection may be transmitted to others.

(2) There occurs generalized lymphadenopathy in the neck, axilla, groin with fever, night sweats and oral thrush.

(3) Further, there is the AIDS related complex with great damage to the immune system accompanied with fatigue, fever, oral thrush, diarrhea and splenomegaly.

(4) Next occurs, full blown AIDS, marked by a collapsing immune system with invasion of life threatening infections, which are usually fatal.

(5) AIDS dementia occurs, when the AIDS virus passes through the blood brain barrier.

Signs and symptoms: Preliminary symptoms are viral illness with low grade fever and chest symptoms leading to pneumonia and even respiratory failure. There is also debilitating dementia; loss of blood vessels (Kaposi's sarcoma) may result in bleeding.

Preventive measures:—

1. There should be regular screening of blood for AIDS virus.
2. The practice of using contaminated syringe needles should be stopped.
3. There should be motivation or change in sex habits.
4. There should be health education about the disease.

(ii) Under-five clinic: Under-five clinic offers a blend of curative, preventive and promotive health services within the resources available in the country, making use of non-professional auxillaries, thus making the services not only economical but also available to a larger proportion of children in the community.

Aims and objectives:—

The aims and objectives of under-five clinic are set out in the symbol or emblem:—

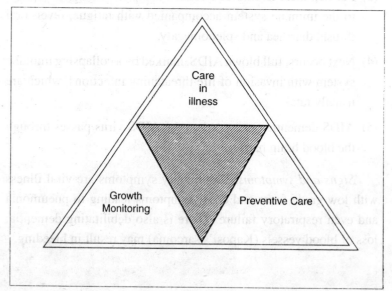

1. Care in illness:—

The apex of the symbol represents "care and treatment of sick children"; care of sick children can be handled by trained nurses.

The illness care for children will comprise of:—

(a) Diagnosis and treatment of:—
   (i) Acute illness.
   (ii) Chronic illness including physical, mental, congenital and acquired abnormalities.
   (iii) Disorders of growth and development.
(b) X-ray and laboratory services.
(c) Referral services.

2. Preventive care:—

(i) Immunization: Of the children against 6 dreadful and preventable diseases. These are diphtheria, tetanus, pertussis, measles, polio, tuberculosis.

(ii) Nutritional surveillance: It is extremely important for identifying sub-clinical nutrition. Almost all major nutritional disorders occurs in this age.

(iii) Health check-ups: Cover physical examination and should be provided every 3 to 6 months.

(iv) Oral rehydration: A poor child suffers 2 to 6 times in a year with diarrhea. The use of ORS has opened the way for a drastic reduction in child mortality and malnutrition.

(v) Family planning: In the center of symbol is a triangular area. If it is colored red we have the family planning triangle of India.

(vi) Health education: Around the whole symbol is a border that touches all areas, this border represents health teachings.

3. Growth monitoring:—

It is to weigh the child periodically at monthly intervals during the first year, every 2 months, during the second year, and every 3 months thereafter up to the age of 5 to 6 years when the child's weight is plotted against his or her age as it gives the *growth curve*.

(iii) Copper T:—

It is a second generation IUD which is smaller and easier to fit.

Advantages of Copper T:—

(a) Low expulsion rate.

(b) Lower incidence of side effects e.g., pain and bleeding.

(c) Easier to fit even in nulliparous women.

(d) Better tolerated by nullipara.

(e) Increased contraceptive effectiveness.

(f) Effective as post-coital contraceptive if inserted 3 to 5 days of unprotected coitus.

Mechanism of action: IUD causes a foreign body reaction in the uterus causing cellular and biochemical changes in the endometrium and uterine fluids which impair viability of the gamete.

Time of insertion: The most appropriate time for loop insertion is during menstruation or within 10 days of beginning of menstrual cycle. During this time, insertion is technically easy because the diameter of cervical canal is greater.

Side effects and complications:—

1. Bleeding.
2. Pain.
3. Pelvic infection.
4. Uterine perforation.
5. Pregnancy.
6. Ectopic pregnancy.
7. Expulsion.
8. Infertility after removal.
9. Cancer and teratogenesis.
10. Mortality.

The ideal IUD candidate:—

(a) Who has borne atleast one child.
(b) Has no history of pelvic disease.
(c) Has normal menstrual periods.
(d) Is willing to check IUD tail.
(e) Has access to follow-up and treatment of potential problems
(f) Is in a monogamous relationship.

Follow-up:—

The objective of follow up is:—

(a) To provide motivation and emotional support for the women.
(b) To confirm the presence of the IUD.
(c) To diagnose and treat any side effects or complications.

II B.H.M.S. 1996

PART A

Q.1 Describe the role of agent, host and environment in causation of disease.

Ans. Natural history of disease: The term natural history of disease signifies the way in which a disease evolves over time from the earliest stage of its prepathogenesis phase to its termination as recovery, disability or death in the absence of treatment or prevention.

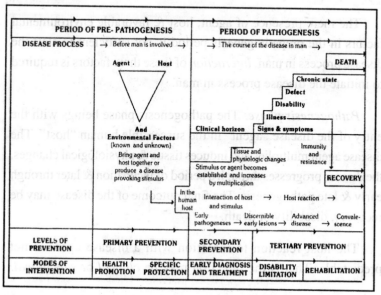

The natural history of disease consists of two phases:—

1. Prepathogenesis phase.
2. Pathogenesis phase.

Prepathogenesis phase: This refers to the period preliminary to the onset of disease in man. The disease agent has not yet entered man; but the factors which favor its interaction with the human host are already existing in the environment.

The causative factors of disease may be classified as:—

(i) Agent.
(ii) Host.
(iii) Environment.

These three factors are referred to as the *epidemiological triad.*

The mere presence of agent, host & favorable environmental factors in the prepathogenesis period is not sufficient to start the disease process in man. *Interaction* of these three factors is required to initiate the disease process in man.

Pathogenesis phase: The pathogenesis phase beings with the entry of the disease "agent" in the susceptible human "host". The disease agent multiplies and induces tissue & physiological changes, the disease progresses through a period of incubation & later through early & late pathogenesis. The final outcome of the disease may be recovery, disability or death.

The host reaction to infection with a disease agent is not predictable. That is the infection may be *clinical* or *subclinical;*

typical or *atypical* or the host may become a carrier with or without developing clinical disease as in case of diphtheria & poliomyelitis.

In chronic diseases (e.g., coronary heart disease, hypertension, cancer), the early pathogenesis phase is less dramatic. This phase in chronic disease is referred to as the presymptomatic phase. During this presymptomatic phase there is no manifest disease. The pathological changes are below "clinical horizon". The clinical stage begins when recognizable signs & symptoms appear.

Levels of prevention:—
1. Primary prevention
2. Secondary prevention.
3. Tertiary prevention.

Primary prevention: It can be defined as action taken prior to the onset of disease, which removes the possibility that disease will ever occur. It signifies the intervention in the prepathogenesis phase or a disease or health problem.

Primary prevention may be accomplished by measures designed to promote general health, well-being & quality of life in people or by specific protective measures.

The WHO has recommended the following approaches for primary prevention of chronic diseases:—

(a) Premordial prevention: Prevention of the emergence or development of risk factors in countries or population groups in which they have not yet appealed. For e.g., smoking, eating patterns.

(b) Population (mass) Strategy: It is directed at the whole population irrespective of individual risk factors. For e.g., studies have shown that even a small reduction in the average blood pressure of a population would produce a large reduction in cardiovascular diseases.

(c) High-risk strategy: It aims to bring preventive care to individuals at special risk. This requires detection of individuals at high risk by optimum use of clinical methods.

Secondary prevention: "Action which halts the progress of a disease at its incipient stage & prevents complications".

The specific interventions are:—

(a) Early diagnosis (e.g., screening tests, case finding programmes).
(b) Adequate treatment.

By early diagnosis and adequate treatment, secondary prevention attempts to arrest the disease process, restore health by seeking out unrecognized disease and treating it before reversible pathological changes have taken place.

3. *Tertiary Prevention:* It signifies intervention in the late pathogenesis phase. Tertiary prevention can be defined as all measures available to reduce or limit impairments and disabilities. For e.g., treatment even if undertaken late in the natural history of a disease may prevent the sequelae and limit disability.

Modes of intervention:—
(i) Health Promotion.
(ii) Specific Protection.
(iii) Early diagnosis and treatment.

(iv) Disability limitation.

(v) Rehabilitation.

(i) *Health promotion:*—It is the process of enabling people to increase control over and to improve health. It is not directed against any particular disease, but is intended to strengthen the host through a variety of approaches (interventions). The well known interventions in this area are:—

(a) Health education.

(b) Environmental modifications.

(c) Nutritional interventions.

(d) Lifestyle and behavioral changes.

(a) Health education: A large number of diseases could be prevented if people are adequately informed about them and if they are encouraged to take necessary precautions in time.

(b) Environmental modifications: Such as provision of safe water; installation of sanitary latrines; control of insects and rodents; improvement of housing, etc.

(c) Nutritional interventions: These comprise of food distribution and nutritional improvement of vulnerable groups, child feeding programmes, food fortifications, nutritional education, etc.

(d) Lifestyle and behavioral changes: The action of prevention in this case is one of individual and community responsibility for health. The physician and each health worker acts as an educator, rather than a therapist.

(ii) *Specific protection:* To avoid disease altogether is the ideal 2but this is possible only in a limited number of cases. The following are some of the currently available interventions aimed at specific protection:—

(a) Immunization.

(b) Use of specific nutrients.

(c) Chemoprophylaxis.

(d) Protection against occupational diseases.

(e) Protection against accidents.

(f) Protection against carcinogens.

(g) Avoidance of allergens.

(h) The control of specific hazards in general environment.

(iii) *Early diagnosis and treatment:* Are main interventions of disease control. The earlier a disease is diagnosed and treated the better it is from the point of view of prognosis and preventing the occurrence of further cases or any longterm disability.

(iv) *Disability limitation:* When a patient reports late in the pathogenesis phase the mode of intervention is disability limitation.

Concept of disability:—

Disease

↓

Impairment

↓

Disability

↓

Handicap

Impairment: Any loss or abnormality of psychological, physiological or anatomical structure or functions.

E.g., loss of foot, defective vision.

Disability: Because of an impairment, the affected person may be unable to carry out certain activities considered normal for his age, sex, etc.

Handicap: It is defined as a disadvantage for a given individual, resulting from an impairment or a disability that limits or prevents the fulfillment of a role that is normal.

(v) *Rehabilitation:* Defined as the combined and coordinated use of medical, social, educational and vocational measures for training and retraining the individual to the highest possible level of functional ability.

Or

What preventive measures will you take in the event of a Gastroenteritis epidemic in the city?

Ans. Chlorination of water: Chlorination is one of the greatest advances in water purification. Various methods of chlorination are:—

(1) *Chlorine gas:* It is cheap, quick in action, efficient and easy to apply. It is applied by a special equipment called chlorinating equipment. It is the method of first choice.

(2) *Chloramines:* Are loose compounds of chlorine and ammonia. They have a less tendency to produce chlorinous taste and give

a more persistent type of residual chlorine. The greatest drawbacks of chloramines is that they have a slower action than chlorine so it is not used to a great extent in water treatment.

(3) *Perchloran:* It is a calcium compound which carries 60-70% of available chlorine.

The following measures will be employed to check gastroenteritis epidemic:—

(1) *Notification:* Early notification is very important. An outbreak of gastroenteritis should be notified immediately by telegram to the district health authority, state and national health authority.

(2) *Isolation of the case:* In the hospital or in the house should be done. The contacts should be segregated and treated.

(3) *Sterilization of water:* The water supplies should be protected from contamination and immediate disinfection of those supplies which are believed to be exposed to risk of pollution. The water may be sterilized by:—

(i) Chlorination

(ii) Permanganate of potash.

(iii) Boiling.

4. *Protection of food:* Food should be well cooked and properly protected from flies, dust, etc. Uncooked food should be avoided and no one should be allowed to handle food without thoroughly washing and disinfecting their hands.

5. *Fly control:* By DDT, malathion spray.

6. *Disposal of night soil:* Indiscrete defections should be avoided or stopped. Quick and effective disposal of night soil should be done, so that flies may not come in contact with night soil.

7. *Disinfection:* Concurrent and terminal disinfection is required. Bleaching powder can be used.

(a) Stools and vomit: All excreta and vomit should be collected in a basin and mixed with an equal quantity of 5% cresol or 3% bleaching powder. After two hours of disinfection it should be burnt or buried.

(b) Clothings and beddings: The cloth should be soaked in 2½% cresol solution for ½ an hour and then washed with soap and water.

(c) Floors and walls: The floor must be thoroughly disinfected with 5% cresol. The walls upto a height of 3 feet should be treated similarly.

(d) Cooking utensils: Disinfected by boiling for 15 minutes or keeping them in cresol solution for ½ hour before washing finally with water and soda.

(e) Hands: Dipped in 1% cresol.

8. *Vaccination.*

9. *Health education.*

Q.2 Discuss the role of breast feeding v/s artificial feeding for a new born baby?

Ans. Breast milk: It is the ideal food for the infant. No other food is required by the baby until 4-5 months after birth.

Advantages of breast milk are:—

(i) If is safe, clean, hygienic, cheap and available to the infant at a correct temperature.

(ii) It meets the nutritional requirements of the infant in the first few months.

(iii) It contains antimicrobial agents such as macrophages, lymphocytes, secretory IgA, anti-streptococcal factor, etc.

(iv) It is easily digested and utilized by both normal and premature babies.

(v) It promotes bonding betweem mother and infant.

(vi) Sucking is good for the baby; for the development of jaw and teeth.

(vii) Protects the baby from a tendency to obesity.

(viii) It prevents malnutrition and reduces infant mortality.

Artificial feeding: The main indications are failure of breast milk, prolonged illness or death of mother.

(a) *Dried milk*: Safest milk prepared scientifically for infant feeding. It is free from bacteria, it does not become sour and it is fortified with vitamins.

(b) *Cow's milk*: Is a cheaper alternative used for infant feeding.

Artificial feeding is a hazardous procedure in poor families because of danger of contamination.

Or

Describe the diarrheal disease control programme in our country.

Ans. Chlorination is one of the greatest advances in water purification. Various methods of chlorination are:—

(1) *Chlorine gas:* It is cheap, quick in action, efficient and easy to apply. It is applied by a special equipment called chlorinating equipment. It is the method of first choice.

(2) *Chloramines:* Are loose compounds of chlorine and ammonia. They have a less tendency to produce chlorinous taste and give a more persistent type of residual chlorine. The greatest drawbacks of chloramines is that they have a slower action than chlorine so it is not used to a great extent in water treatment.

(3) *Perchloran:* It is a calcium compound which carries 60-70% of available chlorine.

The following measures will be employed to check gastroenteritis epidemic:—

(1) *Notification:* Early notification is very important. An outbreak of gastroenteritis should be notified immediately by telegram to the district health authority, state and national health authority.

(2) *Isolation of the case:* In the hospital or in the house should be done. The contacts should be segregated and treated.

(3) *Sterilization of water:* The water supplies should be protected from contamination and immediate disinfection of those supplies which are believed to be exposed to risk of pollution. The water may be sterilized by:—

(i) Chlorination
(ii) Permanganate of potash.
(iii) Boiling.

4. *Protection of food:* Food should be well cooked and properly protected from flies, dust, etc. Uncooked food should be avoided and no one should be allowed to handle food without thoroughly washing and disinfecting their hands.

5. *Fly control:* By DDT, malathion spray.

6. *Disposal of night soil:* Indiscrete defections should be avoided or stopped. Quick and effective disposal of night soil should be done, so that flies may not come in contact with night soil.

7. *Disinfection:* Concurrent and terminal disinfection is required. Bleaching powder can be used.

(a) Stools and vomit: All excreta and vomit should be collected in a basin and mixed with an equal quantity of 5% cresol or 3% bleaching powder. After two hours of disinfection it should be burnt or buried.

(b) Clothings and beddings: The cloth should be soaked in 2½% cresol solution for ½ an hour and then washed with soap and water.

(c) Floors and walls: The floor must be thoroughly disinfected with 5% cresol. The walls upto a height of 3 feet should be treated similarly.

(d) Cooking utensils: Disinfected by boiling for 15 minutes or keeping them in cresol solution for ½ hour before washing finally with water and soda.

(e) Hands: Dipped in 1% cresol.

8. *Vaccination.*

9. *Health education.*

Q.3 Discuss the prevention and control of hookworm infection.

Ans. Diseases transmitted by indiscriminate defecation are:—

(i) Typhoid fever.

(ii) Paratyphoid fever.

(iii) Dysenteries.

(iv) Diarrhea.

(v) Cholera.

(vi) Hookworms.

(vii) Ascariasis.

(viii) Infective hepatitis.

From above it is clear that hookworm is one of these.

Prevention and control of hookworm infection: Prevention and control involves four approaches:—

1. Sanitary disposal of feces.
2. Chemotherapy.
3. Correction of anemia.
4. Health education.

1. *Sanitary technology:* Longterm solution of the problem is the sanitary disposal of human excreta through installation of sewage disposal system in urban areas. This alone will prevent soil pollution.

2. *Chemotherapy:* Periodic case finding and treatment of all

infected persons in the community will reduce the worm burden and frequency of transmission.

3. *Treatment of anemia:* When anemia is severe it should be treated. A cheap and effective treatment is ferrous sulphate 200 mg, three time a day, orally, continued upto 3 months after the Hb has risen to 12 g/100 ml.

4. *Health education:* Community involvement through health education is an important aspect for control of hookworm infection. Health education should be aimed at the use of sanitary latrines and prevention of soil pollution.

Or

Describe the duties of a medical officer posted in a festival.

Ans. Sanitary measures are:—

1. *Before the mela:—*

(a) Selection of site: The health officer and district engineer should go to the fair site for selection of site and preparation of the necessary programme for lodging houses, proper conservancy, water supply, general sanitation and the required equipment. Roads should be marked and repaired.

(b) General arrangement: All necessary materials like brooms, strings, lime and bleaching powder should be stored in godowns.

(c) Staff required and materials:—

(i) Medical officer – one.

(ii) Health inspector – one.

(iii) One sweeper for every 1000 people for trench latrine.

    (iv) One sweeper for every 5000 person per day for picking up from the road.

    (v) One sweeper for every 2000 person per day for collecting rubbish and dumping it.

    (vi) Some extra sweepers dealing with other urgent matters.

    (vii) Disinfectants.

(d) Water supply: Adequate and safe water supply is of utmost important.

(e) Refuse and conservancy system: Bore hole latrines are very suitable and hygienic for the purpose. It must reach 1 feet below the sub-soil water. Dustbins, urinals and soakage pits etc. should be provided at suitable places.

2. *During the mela:—*

(a) Water Supply: Wells should be regularly disinfected. If water has been found unfit for drinking, it should be made undrinkable by pouring kerosene oil on them, or keeping a watch so that nobody drinks that unfit water. Water should be drawn by special men with proper buckets. Inspecting staff should have test tubes, potassium iodide crystals and starch powder to test the presence of chlorine and to know whether the wells have been disinfected properly or not.

(b) Refuse disposal: The refuse and road sweepings should be disposed off properly.

(c) Conservancy: Male and female latrines should be marked. They should be lighted during the night. Sweepers should be posted at each latrine for cleaning and filling the used latrine. Bleaching powder and lime should be sprinkled freely. People should be prevented from passing stool on the ground.

(d) Food sanitation: The sale of stale food, unripe and over-ripe fruits should not be permitted. One medical officer should be authorized to seize any unwholesome articles of food and destroy the same.

(e) Accommodation: There should not be over-crowding in rooms; sick people should be moved to the hospital.

(f) Medical care: Dispensaries should be under a competent medical officer. Arrangement for emergencies should be made.

PART B

Q.4 What precautions will you take in the disposal of a body of an AIDS patient? How will you declare the premises fit for human living after the death of the patient in a government accommodation?

Ans. The precautions are as follows:—

(i) The articles used by the patient should be disinfected.

(ii) The patient's urine, feces, sputum should be properly disinfected.

(iii) Proper sterlization of instruments should be enforced.

Or

What treatment will you administer to a patient bitten by:—

(i) Dog.

(ii) Monkey.

(iii) **Camel.**

(iv) **Cow.**

Ans. Dog, monkey, camel and cow are all warm-blooded animals. They transmit the zoonotic disease *Rabies* to man by their bites if they are rabid.

The *causative* agent of rabies is a bullet shaped neurotropic RNA containing virus. The transfer of infection from wild life to domestic animals results in creation of urban cycle.

The *source of infection* to man is the saliva of rabid animals.

Treatment:—

There is no specific treatment for rabies, Case management includes the following procedure:—

(a) The patient should be isolated in a quiet soon protected as far as possible from stimuli such as bright light, noise or cold draughts which may precipitate spasms or convulsions.

(b) Relieve anxiety and pain by liberal use of sedatives. Morphia in doses of 30-45 mg may be given repeatedly. The drug is well tolerated and once the diagnosis is established there appears to be no reason to restrict the administration of a drug which does so much to allay acute suffering.

(c) If spastic muscular contractions are present, use drugs with curare-like action.

(d) Ensure hydration and diuresis.

(e) Intensive therapy in the form of respiratory and cardiac support may be given.

Prevention of rabies:—

1. Post-exposure prophylaxis:—

    (a) Cleansing: Immediate flushing and washing the wounds, scratches and the adjoining areas with plenty of soap and water preferably under a running tap for at least 5 minutes is of paramount importance. In case of punctured wounds catheters, should be used to irrigate the wounds.

    (b) Chemical treatment: Whatever residual virus remains in the wound after cleansing should be inactivated by irrigation with viricidal agents, either alcohol, tincture, aq. solution of iodine.

    (c) Suturing: Bite wounds should not be immediately sutured to prevent additional trauma.

    (d) Antirabies serum.

    (e) Antibiotics and anti-tetanus serum.

    (f) Observe the animal for 10 days: Observe the biting animal for at least 10 days from the day of bite. If the animal shows symptom of rabies, it should be humanely killed and its head is removed and sent for FRA test.

2. Immunization: Human anti-rabies vaccination.

Technique of administration: Ideal site for vaccination is the anterior abdominal wall, for this area offers enough space to accommodate the large quantity of vaccine to be injected. The area is divided into quadrants and a different site is used for each injection.

To ensure proper administration, a fold of skin is lifted between the thumb and other fingers with the patient in a lying down or standing position.

Q.5 Name the diseases spread by arthropods. Describe the control measures for any one of them.

Ans.

	Arthropod	Diseases transmitted
1.	Mosquito	- Malaria - Filaria - Dengue
2.	Housefly	- Typhoid - Diarrhea - Cholera - Amoebiasis - Conjunctivitis - Trachoma
3.	Sand-fly	- Kala-azar - Oriental sore - Sand-fly fever
4.	Tsetse fly	- Sleeping sickness
5.	Louse	- Epidemic typhus - Relapsing fever - Trench fever
6.	Rat flea	- Bubonic plague - Endemic typhus
7.	Reduvid bug	- Chagas disease
8.	Hard tick	- Tick typhus

		- Viral encephalitis
		- Viral fevers
9.	Soft tick	Q fever.
		- Relapsing fever.

Control measure of filaria:—

The prevention is based on:—

(a) Chemotherapy.

(b) Vector control.

Chemotherapy: Action of drugs against microfilariae and the adult worms in human host.

Vector control: Mosquito Control Measures.

1. *Anti-larval measures:—*

(a) Environmental control: Reducing their breeding places. This is known as source reduction and comprises of minor engineering methods such as filling, leveling and drainage of breeding places:—

Culex: Reducing domestic and predomestic sources of breeding such as cesspools and open ditches.

Aedes: Environment should be cleaned up and got rid of water holding containers such as discarded tins, empty pots, broken bottles, etc.

Anopheles: Breeding places should be looked for and abolished by appropriate engineering measures.

Mansonia: Reduce the aquatic plants.

(b) Chemical control: Commonly used larvicides are:—

    (i) Mineral oils.

    (ii) Paris green.

    (iii) Synthetic insecticides.

Mineral oils: The application of oil to water is one of the oldest known mosquito control measures. Since the life cycle of a mosquito occupies about 8 days or so it is customary to apply oil once a week on all breeding places.

Paris green: It is a stomach poison and to be effective it must be ingested by the larvae. Anopheles are surface feeders so it is easily killed by Paris green and for bottom feeders Paris green is applied in granular formation.

Synthetic insecticides: E.g., fenthion, chlorpyrifos and abate are effective larvicides. These organophosphorus compounds hydrolyze quickly in water.

(c) Biological control: A wide range of small fish feed readily on mosquito larvae. The best known are Gambusia offense and Lebister reticulatus.

2. *Anti-adult measures:*—

(a) Residual sprays: E.g., DDT 1-2 grams of pure DDT per sq. metre are applied 3 times a year to walls and other surfaces where mosquitoes rest.

(b) Space sprays: These are those where the insecticidal formulation is sprayed into the atmosphere in the form of mist or fog to kill insects.

Common space sprays are:—

(i) Pyrethrum extract: Pyrethrum flowers form an excellent space sprays.

It has the active principle *pyrethrin* which is a nerve poison and kills the insects instantly on mere contact.

(ii) Residual insecticide: Malathion and jenitrothin.

(c) Genetic control:—
- (i) Sterile male technique.
- (ii) Cytoplasmic incompatibility.
- (iii) Chromosomal translocations.
- (iv) Sex distortion.
- (v) Gene replacement.

3. *Protection against mosquito bites:—*

(a) Mosquito net: It offers protection against mosquito bites during sleep. The net should be white to allow easy detection of mosquitoes. Best pattern is a rectangular net.

The size of opening should not exceed 0.0475 inch in diameter. The number of holes in one square inch are usually 150.

(b) Screening: Of buildings with copper or bronze gauze having 16 meshes to the inch is recommended. The aperture should not be larger than 0.0475 inch.

(c) Repellents: Like Diethyl toluamide is active against fatigans.

Or

Describe the methods of chlorination of:—

(i) Overhead water tank of a colony.

(ii) Well.

(iii) Swimming pool.

(iv) Earthern pot.

Ans. Overhead water tank of the colony: It is purified by chlorination. We use chlorine tablets which come under the trade name of "Halazone Tablets".

They are quite good for disinfecting small quantities of water. "Chlorine demand" of the water should be estimated. The chlorine demand of water is the difference between the amount of chlorine added to the water and the amount of residual chlorine remaining at the end of the specific period of contact (usually 60 minutes) at a given temperature and pH of water. The point at which the chlorine demand of water is met is called "break point". Then we test free residual chlorine which should be 0.5 mg/l for one hour.

(ii) Well:—

They are the main sources of water supply in the rural areas. Steps in well disinfections are as follows:—

(1) Find the volume of water in a well.

    (a) Measure the depth of water column = (h) metre.

    (b) Measure the diameter of well = (d) metre.

$$\text{Volume (litres)} = \frac{3.14 \times d^2 \times h}{4} \times 1000$$

(2) Roughly 2.5 grams of good quality bleaching powder would be required to disinfect 1,000 litres of water.

(3) The bleaching powder required for disinfecting the well is placed in a bucket and made into a thin paste. More water is added till the bucket is nearly ¾th full. The contents are stirred well and allowed to sediment for 5 to 10 minutes. When the lime settles down, the supernatant solution which is a chlorine solution is transferred to another bucket and the chalk or lime is discarded.

(4) The bucket containing the chlorine solution is lowered some distance below the water surface and the well water is agitated by moving the bucket violently both vertically and laterally. This should be done several times so that the chlorine solution mixes intimately with the water inside the well.

(5) Contact period should be 1 hour.

(6) Free residual chlorine should be 0.5 mg/litre in the 1st hour.

(iii) Swimming pool:—

Water is exposed to:—

(a) Fecal contamination.

(b) Organisms from skin and naso-pharynx.

Chlorination is the most widely used method of pool disinfection. Various workers have stated that a continuous maintenance of 1.0 mg/litre of free chlorine residual provides an adequate protection against bacterial and viral agents. The pH of water is kept between 7.4-7.8.

(iv) Earthen pot:—

Water can be chlorinated by bleaching powder; it contains 33% available chlorine.

Q.6 What sanitary measures will you advice for a rural area in respect of house building and maintenance of sufficient cross-ventilation?

Ans. In the rural areas the minimum standards of house building are:—

1. There should be at least two living rooms.
2. Ample verandah space may be provided.
3. The built up area should not exceed one third of the total area.
4. There should be a separate kitchen with a paved sink or plateform for washing utensils.
5. The house should be provided with a sanitary latrine.
6. The window area should be at least 10% of the floor area.
7. There should be a sanitary well or a tubewell within a quarter of a mile from the house.
8. It is insanitary to keep cattle and livestock in dwelling houses.

Ventilation: Ventilation means the constant replacement of foul air by fresh air through inlets and outlets. It also means the control of incoming air with regards to its temperature, humidity and purity.

The ventilation can be maintained by:—

(a) Ventilators.
(b) Doors.
(c) Windows.

The ventilation is maintained by:—

Wind: Blowing freely through a room from one side to the other as a result of natural movement.

Diffusion: Means mixing of two types of gases, when doors and windows are closed, air passes out or comes in through cracks in the walls, bricks, windows, etc.

Inequality of temperature: Temperature inequality inside and outside the room. Air flows from high density to low density, it rises when slightly heated; air escapes from openings provided high up in the room. The outside air is cooler and more dense, hence it will enter the rooms through inlets placed low. The greater the temperature differences between outside and inside air, the greater the velocity of the incoming air.

These properties are utilized to the best advantage by proper location of doors, windows, ventilators, etc.

Or

Describe the method to control the rodents in your locality.

Ans. Antirodent measures:—

1. *Sanitation measures*: The environmental sanitation measures comprise of:—

(a) Proper storage, collection and disposal of garbage.

(b) Proper storage of food stuffs.

(c) Construction of rat proof buildings, godowns and warehouses.

(d) Elimination of rat burrows by blocking them with concrete.

2. *Trapping*: It is a simple operation, but it causes temporary reduction in the number of commensal rodents. It is recommended that the number of traps laid should be at least 5% of the human population. The traps are usually baited by food.

3. *Rodenticides*: These are of two types: single dose (acute), lethal to rat after single feeding and multiple dose, which requires repeated feedings over 3 or more days. The commonly used poisons are:—

(i) Barium carbonate: A white tasteless powder which is very cheap. It is mixed with wheat or rice flour in the ratio 1 part to 4 parts of flour. The mixed material is moistened with water and made into small round marbles. The poisoned baits are placed near the rat burrows. On eating the pills the rat is killed within 2 to 24 hours.

(ii) Zinc phosphate: It is an efficient rodenticide when moist. The chemical slowly gives off phosphine whose garlic odor is like a repellent to man and domestic animals. It is used in the ratio of 1 part to 10 part of wheat or rice flour. It may be mixed with a few drops of edible oils in order to render it more attractive to rats.

4. *Fumigation*: An effective method of destroying both rats and rat fleas. The fumigants used are calcium cyanide (cyanogas), carbon disulfide, methyl bromide, SO_2, etc. This chemical is prepared in powder form and is pumped into rat burrow by a special foot pump called the "cyanogas pump". About 2 ounces of the poison are pumped into each rat burrow after closing the exit opening and the burrow is then promptly sealed with wet mud. On contact with moisture, the cyanogas powder gives off hydrogen cyanide gas which is lethal to both rats and their fleas.

5. *Chemosterilants*: It is a chemical that can cause temporary or permanent sterility in either sex or both sexes.

PART C

Q.7 Describe the Universal Immunization Programme with special emphasis on cold chain.

Ans. In May 1974, the WHO officially launched a global immunization programme, known as the Expanded Programme on Immunization (EPI) to protect all children from six vaccine preventable diseases namely:—

(a) Diphtheria.
(b) Whooping cough.
(c) Tetanus.
(d) Polio.
(e) Tuberculosis.
(f) Measles.

The programme is now called Universal Immunization Programme.

Beneficiaries	Age	Vaccine	No. of Doses	Route of Administration
Infants	6 weeks to	DPT	3	Intra muscular
		Polio	3	Oral
	9 months.	BCG	1*	Intra dermal
	9 to 12 months	Measles		Subcutaneous
Children	16 to 24 months	DPT	1**	Intra muscular
		Polio	1**	Oral
	5 to 6	DT	1*	Intra muscular

	years	Typhoid	2	Subcutaneous
	10 years	Tetanus toxoid	1@	Intra muscular
			1@	Subcutaneous
	16 years	Tetanus toxoid	1@	Intra muscular
		Typhoid	1@	Subcutaneous
Pregnant women	16 to 36 weeks	Tetanus toxoid	1@	Intra muscular

*For institutional delivery.

**Booster doses

@ 2 doses, it not vaccinated.

Cold chain: The cold chain is a system of storage and transport of vaccines at low temperature from the manufacturer to the actual vaccination site. The cold chain system is necessary because vaccine failure may occur due to a failure in storing and transporting the vaccine under strict temperature controls. The cold chain equipment consist of:—

(i) Cold box: It is meant to transport large quantities of vaccine by vehicle to out of reach sites.

(ii) Vaccine carrier: It is meant to transport small quantities of vaccine by bicycle or by foot.

(iii) Flasks: They are used if vaccine carriers are not available.

(iv) Ice-packs.

(v) Refrigerator.

Or

What do you understand by antenatal care? Describe in detail the role of Medical Officer and Pubic Health Nurse posted at a PHC in providing MCH services.

Ans. Antenatal are: Antenatal care is the care of the woman during pregnancy. The primary aim of antenatal care is to achieve at the end of pregnancy a healthy mother and a healthy baby.

Objectives:—

1. To promote, protect and maintain the health of the mother during pregnancy.
2. To detect "high risk" cases and give them special attention.
3. To foresee complications and prevent them.
4. To remove anxiety and dread associated with delivery.
5. To reduce maternal and infant mortality and morbidity.
6. To teach the mother elements of childcare, nutrition, personal hygiene and environmental sanitation.
7. To sensitize mother to the need of family planning.

Role of a Medical Officer and a Public Health Nurse posted at PHC are:—

1. *Antenatal visits:* Once a month during the first 7 months, twice for a next 2 month. Every week thereafter.

Preventive services for mother:—

A. At first visit:—

(i) Health history.
(ii) Physical examination.
(iii) Laboratory examination.
    (a) Complete urine analysis.
    (b) Stool examination.
    (c) Complete blood count.

(d) Serological examinations.

(e) Blood grouping and Rh estimation.

(f) Chest X-ray if needed.

(g) Pap test.

(h) G.C. culture.

B. On subsequent visits:—

(i) Physical examination (eg., weight gain, B.P.).

(ii) Lab test (urine and Hb estimation).

(iii) Fe and folic acid supplementation.

(iv) Immunization against tetanus.

(v) Group or individual instructions on nutrition, family planning, self-care, delivery, etc.

(vi) Home visiting.

Maintenance of record: Every woman has her own antenatal card (ANC):

2. *Prenatal advice:* A major component of antenatal care is antenatal advice.

(i) Diet: Pregnancy in total duration consumes about 60,000 Kcal over and above normal metabolic requirements. On an average, there is 12 kg weight gain during pregnancy. So the pregnant woman should take a balanced and adequate diet.

(ii) Personal hygiene:—

(a) Personal cleanliness: She should bathe everyday and wear clean clothes.

    (b) Rest and sleep: 8 hours sleep and at least 2 hours rest after mid day meal.

    (c) Bowels: Constipation should be avoided by regular intake of green leafy vegetables.

    (d) Exercise: Light exercise.

    (e) No smoking.

    (f) Maintain oral hygiene.

    (g) Sexual intercourse should be restricted during pregnancy.

(iii) Drugs: She should not take any drugs without the doctor.

(iv) Radiation: No X-rays should be done during pregnancy.

(v) Warning signs: Mother should be given clear cut instructions that she should immediately report when:—

    (a) Swelling of feet.

    (b) Fits.

    (c) Headache.

    (d) Blurring of vision.

    (e) Bleeding per vagina.

    (f) Any other unusual symptoms.

(vi) Child care: Advice on hygiene and child rearing.

(vii) Family planning.

(viii) Immunization against tetanus.

    Diet of a pregnant woman:—

    The pregnancy diet should be light, nutritious, easily digestible and rich in protein, minerals and vitamins. The diet should consist of principal foods along with one litre of milk, one egg, plenty of green vegetables and fruits. At least, half of the total protein should be first class and the majority of fat should be animal type. Supplementary iron therapy is needed for all pregnant mothers, 1 tablet daily of ferrous sulphate complaining 60 mg of elemental iron.

Recommended daily nutrients for a pregnant woman:—

Kilocalories	2500
Protein	60 gm
Calcium	1000 mg
Iron	40 mg
Vitamin A	6000 IU
Vitamin D	400 IU
Thiamine	1.5 mg
Riboflavine	1.5 mg
Nicotinic acid	15 mg
Ascorbic acid	60 mg
Folic acid	1 mg
Vitamin B_{12}	2µg

3. *Specific health protection:—*

(i) Anemia: 60 mg of elemental iron and 500 mcg of folic acid in one tablet is given every day to pregnant mothers.

(ii) Nutritional deficiencies: To protect the mother from vitamin and protein deficiency, fresh milk or skimmed milk is given in MCH centers. Capsules of Vitamin A and D are also supplied.

(iii) **Toxemias of pregnancy:** Early detection and management of albumin in urine and an increase in B.P.

(iv) **Tetanus:** If the mother is not immunized earlier, 2 doses of absorbed tetanus toxoid should be given; Ist dose at 16-20 weeks. IInd dose is given at 20-24 weeks of pregnancy; the third dose is given 1 month before the expected date of delivery.

(v) **Syphilis:** Test blood for syphilis. Congenital syphilis can be prevented by ten daily injections of procaine penicillin.

(vi) **German measles:** If the mother suffers from German measles during the first trimester, the infant may have congenital abnormalities. In such cases, termination of pregnancy may be considered.

(vii) **Rh status:** In order to prevent Rh sensitization in all women at risk, intramuscular administration of 200 to 300 µg of Rh immunoglobulin at 28 and 34 weeks with a further dose after delivery if the baby is Rh positive.

4. *Mental preparation:* Of mother for delivery.

5. *Family planning:* Mother should be given advice for family planning, to have a secure, good and happy life.

Q.8 Describe the methods taken by government to control environmental pollution in Delhi.

Ans. **Methods taken by government to control air pollution are:—**

1. *Containment:* Prevention of escape of toxic substances into the ambient air. Containment can be achieved by a variety of engineering methods such as enclosure, ventilation and air cleaning.

2. *Replacement:* This is replacing a technological process

causing air pollution by a new process that does not cause any pollution.

3. *Dilution:* Is valid so long as it is within the self leaning capacity of the environment. The establishment of "green belts" between industrial and residential areas is an attempt at dilution.

4. *Legislation:* Many countries have adopted legislation for control of air pollution.

5. *International action:* To deal with air pollution on a world wide scale, the WHO has established an international network of laboratories for the monitoring and study of air pollution.

The Govt. is converting the diesel buses into CNG which is environment friendly. Aslo, Metro Rail Project is being completed at a very high speed, which will decongest the roads and make the air of Delhi more clean. Also, all the pollution causing factories have been shifted out of Delhi. Many flyovers have been built so that the vehicles spend less time on red lights which causes pollution.

Or

Q.8 Discuss the Pulse Polio Immunization programme.

Ans. The Pulse Polio Immunization Programme was started by the government of India.

In this programme, all the children upto 5 years of age are given oral polio vaccine by the domiciliary workers. In the beginning the programme was conducted in November, December and January at various centres. But in the year 2000 it was conducted in 4 months in the danger areas i.e. in September also. This year house to house duties were also given to workers so that we can achieve complete immunization.

The vaccine should be stored in a deep freeze. The vaccine is provided to various centres in a vaccine carrier in which ice cubes are present along with the vaccine. Two drops are put in the mouth of the child. Vaccinators use droppers supplied with the vial of OPV. This is the most direct and effective way to deliver the correct drop size. Tilt the child's back, and gently squeeze the cheeks or pinch the nose to make their mouth open. Let the, drops fall from the dropper on to the child's tongue. On administration, the live vaccine infects the intestinal epithelial cells.

The virus after replication is transported to Peyer's patches where a secondary multiplication occurs. The virus spreads to other parts of the body resulting in the production of circulating antibodies which prevent dissemination of the virus to the nervous system and prevent paralytic polio. Intestinal infection stimulates the production of IgA secretary antibodies which prevent subsequent infection of the alimentary tract.

Advantages of OPV:—

(i) Since it is given orally, it can be administered by domiciliary workers.

(ii) Induces both humoral and intestinal immunity.

(iii) Inexpensive.

(iv) Useful in controlling epidemics.

Q.9 Write short notes on:—

(i) IMR.

(ii) Mean, Mode Median.

(iii) Incidence and Prevalence.

Ans. (i) IMR:—

It is defined as the ratio of infant deaths registered in a given year to the total number of live births registered in the same year, usually expressed as a rate per 1000 live births.

$$IMR = \frac{\text{Number of deaths of children less than 1yr of age in a year}}{\text{Number of live births in the same year}} \times 1000$$

(ii) Mean, Mode, Median:—

Mean: To obtain a mean, the individual observations are first added together and then divided by the number of observation.

The operation of adding together is called "summation" denoted by sign Σ. Mean is denoted by x.

Advantages: Easy to calculate and understand.

Disadvantages: Sometimes it may be unduly influenced by abnormal values in the distribution.

Median: The median is an average of a different kind, which does not depend upon the total and number of items. To obtain the median the data is first arranged in the ascending or descending order of magnitude and then the value of the middle observation is located which is called the median.

Mode: It is the commonly occurring value in a distribution of data. It is the most frequent item or the most "fashionable" value in a series of observation.

Advantages:—

(a) The advantages of mode are that it is easy to understand.

(b) It is not affected by the extreme items.

Disadvantages: The exact location is often uncertain and is often not clearly defined.

(iii) Incidence and Prevalence:—

Incidence: Incidence rate is defined as the number of new cases occurring in a defined population during a specified period of time.

$$\frac{\text{Number of new cases of specific disease during a given time period}}{\text{Population at risk}} \times 1000$$

Incidence refers:—

(a) Only to new cases.

(b) During a given period of time.

(c) In a specified population or population at risk.

(d) It can also refer to new spells or episodes of disease arising in a given period of time per 1000 population.

Uses of incidence rate: The incidence rate as a health status indicated is useful for taking action:—

(a) To control disease.

(b) For search into etiology and pathogenesis, distribution of diseases and efficacy of preventive and therapeutic measures.

Prevalence: It is of two types:—

(a) Point prevalence.

(b) Period prevalence.

(a) Point prevalence: If a disease is defined as the number of all current cases (old and new) of disease at one point in time in relation to a defined population.

Point prevalence is given by the formula:—

$$\frac{\text{Number of all current cases (old and new) of a specified disease existing at a given point in time}}{\text{Estimated population at the same point in time}} \times 100$$

Point prevalence can be made specific for age, sex and other relevant factors or attributes.

(b) Period prevalence: A less commonly used measure of prevalence is period prevalence. It measures the frequency of all current cases existing during a defined period of time expressed in relation to a defined population. It includes cases arising before but extending into or through the year as well as those cases arising during the year.

Period prevalence is given by following formula:—

$$\frac{\text{Number of existing cases of a specified disease during a given period of time interval}}{\text{Estimated mid-interval population at risk}} \times 100$$

Relationship between prevalence and incidence:—

Prevalence depends upon 2 factors, the incidence and duration of illness.

$$P = I \times D$$
$$= \text{Incidence} \times \text{Mean duration.}$$

Uses of prevalence:—

(a) Prevalence helps to estimate the magnitude of health/disease problems in the community and identify potential high risk populations.

(b) Prevalence rates are especially useful for administrative and planning purposes.

II B.H.M.S. 1997

PART A

Q.1 Define health. State the relation of economic and environmental factors to health and disease?

Ans. Health is a state of complete physical, mental and social well-being and not merely an absence of disease or infirmity.

Health and disease are both related to environment eg., climate, water, air, etc.

Environment is classified as internal and external. The internal environment of man pertains to "each and every component part, every tissue, organ and organ system and their harmonious functioning within the system." Internal environment is the domain of the internal machine.

The external or macro-environment consists of those things to which man is exposed to after conception. It is defined as "all that which is external to individual human host." It can be divided into:—

(a) Physical
(b) Biological
(c) Psychosocial components

Any or all of which can affect the health of man and his susceptibility to illness.

"Micro environment" term used as personal environment to which includes the individual's way of living and lifestyle, e.g. eating habits, smoking, etc.

It is established that environment has a direct impact on the physical, mental and social wellbeing of those living in it. The environmental factors range from – housing, water supply, psychosocial stress and family structure through social and economic support systems to the organization of health and social welfare services in the community.

If the environment is favorable to the individual, he can make full use of his physical and mental capabilities.

(i) Economic status: The per capita GNP is the most widely accepted measure of general economic performance. It is the economic progress that has been the major factor in reducing morbidity, increasing life expectancy and improving the quality of life.

The economic status determines the purchasing power, standard of living, quality of life, family size and pattern of disease and deviant behavior in the community. It is also an important factor in seeking health care.

(ii) Education: A second major factor influencing health status is education. The world map of illiteracy closely coincides with maps of poverty, malnutrition, ill health, high infant and child mortality rates.

(iii) Occupation: The very state of being employed in productive works promotes health because the unemployed usually show a higher incidence of ill health and death.

(iv) Political system: Health is also related to the country's political system.

Q.2 Describe the etiology, clinical presentation, complications and prevention of chickenpox.

Ans. *Causative organism:* Varicella zoster or V-Z. It is a filterable virus related to the herpes zoster virus.

Incubation period: 14 to 16 days.

Source of infection: Infected persons.

Mode of spread: Droplet infection.

Clinical features:—

1. The infection is of sudden onset accompanied by mild fever and itching. This prodromal phase usually lasts for a day or so.
2. It is followed by eruptions, which occur as macules, papules, vesicles and pustule formations occurring in quick succession.
3. The eruption phase lasts for about 4-5 days.

Complications: Are rare but these can occur.

(a) Pneumonia.
(b) Encephalitis.

The disease confers life long immunity.

Prevention: No specific active immunization is available.

Q.3 What do you understand by cold chain? What is the role of a general medical practitioner in the National Immunization Programme?

Ans. In May 1974, the WHO officially launched a global immunization programme, known as the Expanded Programme on Immunization (EPI) to protect all children from six vaccine preventable diseases namely:—

(a) Diphtheria.
(b) Whooping cough.
(c) Tetanus.
(d) Polio.
(e) Tuberculosis.
(f) Measles.

The programme is now called Universal Immunization Programme.

Beneficiaries	Age	Vaccine	No. of Doses	Route of Administration
Infants	6 weeks to 9 months. 9 to 12 months	DPT Polio BCG Measles	3 3 1*	Intra muscular Oral Intra dermal Subcutaneous
Children	16 to 24 months 5 to 6 years 10 years 16 years	DPT Polio DT Typhoid Tetanus toxoid Tetanus toxoid Typhoid	1** 1** 1* 2 1@ 1@ 1@ 1@	Intra muscular Oral Intra muscular Subcutaneous Intra muscular Subcutaneous Intra muscular Subcutaneous
Pregnant women	16 to 36 weeks	Tetanus toxoid	1@	Intra muscular

*For institutional delivery.
**Booster doses
@ 2 doses, it not vaccinated.

Cold chain: The cold chain is a system of storage and transport of vaccines at low temperature from the manufacturer to the actual vaccination site. The cold chain system is necessary because vaccine failure may occur due to a failure in storing and transporting the vaccine under strict temperature controls. The cold chain equipment consist of:—

(i) Cold box: It is meant to transport large quantities of vaccine by vehicle to out of reach sites.

(ii) Vaccine carrier: It is meant to transport small quantities of vaccine by bicycle or by foot.

(iii) Flasks: They are used if vaccine carriers are not available.

(iv) Ice-packs.

(v) Refrigerator.

Role of GMP: As the general medical practitioner is the person who is very near in a said community, therefore, he has a great role to play in the National Immunization Programme. The most important role of GMP is to create awareness among his clientele about the various diseases which can be prevented by immunization. Also, he has to motivate his patients to get immunized as early as possible.

PART B

Q.4 How can water be purified for drinking purposes? Describe the methods that can be used at small scale. (6)

Ans. Water can be purified for drinking purposes by:—

1. Storage.
2. Filtration.
3. Chlorination.

1. Storage: Water is drawn out from the source and impounded in natural or artificial reservoirs. Storage provides a reserve of water from which further pollution is excluded. As a result of storage, a very considerable amount of purification takes place by:—

(a) *Physical process*: 90% impurities settle down due to gravity. The water becomes clearer.

(b) *Chemical*: The aerobic bacteria oxidize the organic matter present in the water with the aid of dissolved oxygen.

(c) *Biological*: A tremendous drop takes place in bacterial count during storage.

2. Filtration: It is the second stage in the purification of water and quite an important stage because 98-99% of bacteria are removed by filtration.

3. Chlorination: It is one of the greatest advances in water purification. It is a supplement and not a substitute to sand filtration. Chlorine kills pathogenic bacteria but it has no effect on spores and certain viruses (e.g., polio, viral hepatitis).

Principles of chlorination:—

1. First of all, the water to be chlorinated should be clear and free from turbidity. Turbidity impedes efficient chlorination.
2. Secondly, the "chlorine demand" of water is to be estimated. The chlorine demand of water is the difference between the amount of chlorine added to the water and the amount of residual chlorine remaining at the end of a specific period of contact (usually 60 minutes) at a given temperature and pH of the water. The point at which the chlorine demand of water is met is called the "break point".
3. Contact period should be at least one hour.

The minimum recommended concentration of free chlorine is 0.5 mg/l for one hour.

Purification of water on a small scale:—

1. *Household purification of water:—*

Three methods are generally available for purifying water on a small scale. These methods can be used singly or in combination.

(a) Boiling: Boiling is a satisfactory method of purifying water for household purposes. To be effective the water must be brought to a "rolling boil" for 5 to 10 minutes. It kills all bacteria, spores, cysts and ova and yields sterilized water. Boiling also removes temporary hardness by driving off CO_2 and precipitating the calcium carbonate. Taste of water is altered. While boiling is an excellent method of purification, it offers no "residual protection" against subsequent microbial contamination. Water should be boiled in the same container in which it is to be stored to avoid contamination during storage.

(b) Clinical disinfections:—

(i) Bleaching powder: It is a white amorphous powder with a pungent smell of chlorine when freshly made. It contains 33% "available chlorine". It is however an unstable compound.

On exposure to light, air it looses its chlorine content. But when mixed with excess of lime, it retains its strength, this is called "stabilized lime."

(ii) Chlorine solution: May be prepared from bleaching powder. If 4 kgs of bleaching powder with 25% available chlorine is mixed with 20 litres of water it will give 5% solution of chlorine.

(iii) High test hypochlorite: These are calcium compounds which contains 60-70% available chlorine. It is more stable than bleaching powder and deteriorates much less on storage.

(iv) Chlorine tablets: These are available in the market under various trade-names (viz. halozone tablets). They are quite good for disinfecting small quantities of water.

(v) Iodine: Two drops of 2% ethanol solution of iodine will suffice for one litre of clear water. A contact time of 20 to 30 minutes is needed for effective disinfections.

(vi) Potassium permanganate: Although a powerful oxidizing agent, it is not a satisfactory agent for disinfecting water. It may kill cholera vibrios, but is of little use against other disease organisms. It alters the color, smell and taste of water.

(c) Filteration:—

Water can be purified on a small scale by filtering through ceramic filters such as Pasteur Chamberland filter, Berkefeld filter

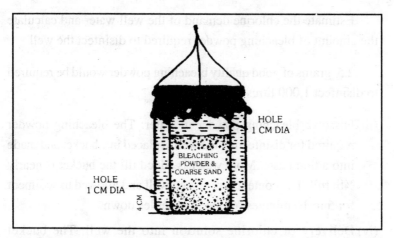

and Katadyn filter. The essential part of filter is the "candle" which is made of porcelain in the Chamberland type and of kieselgurh in the Berkefeld filter.

2. *Disinfection of wells:*—

The most effective and cheapest method of disinfecting wells is by bleaching powder.

Steps in well disinfection:—

(i) Find the volume of water in the well.

    (a) Measure the depth of water column —— (h) meter

    (b) Measure the diameter of well —— (d) metres

    (c) Substitute h and d in

$$V = \frac{3.14 \times d^2 \times h}{4} \times 100$$

    (d) One cubic metre = 1000 litres of water.

(ii) Find the amount of bleaching powder required for disinfection.

Estimate the chlorine demand of the well water and calculate the amount of bleaching powder required to disinfect the well.

2.5 grams of good quality bleaching powder would be required to disinfect 1,000 litres of water.

(iii) Dissolve bleaching powder in water: The bleaching powder required for disinfecting the well is placed in a bucket and made into a thin paste. More water is added till the bucket is nearly ¾th full. The contents are stirred well and allowed to sediment for 5 to 10 minutes for the lime settles down.

(iv) Delivery of chlorine solution into the well. The bucket containing the chlorine solution is lowered some distance below the water surface and the well water is agitated by moving the bucket violently both vertically and laterally.

(v) Contact period should be 1 hour.

(vi) Ortho-tolicline Arsenite Test.

It is a good practice to test for residual chlorine at the end of one hour contact. If the free chlorine level is less than 0.5 mg/litre, the chlorination procedure should be repeated.

Q.5 Define growth and development. How will you assess the growth and development of children below 5 years of age.

Ans. Growth refers to an increase in the physical size of the body.

Development refers to an increase in skill and function. Growth and development are considered together because the child grows and develops as a whole.

In nutritional surveys, the examination of a random and

representative sample of the population covering all ages and both sex in different socio-economic groups is sufficient to be able to draw valid conclusions.

Assessment methods:—

1. Clinical examination.
2. Anthropometry.
3. Biochemical evaluation.
4. Functional assessment.
5. Assessment of dietary intake.
6. Vital and health statistics.
7. Ecological studies.

1. *Clinical examination:* It is an essential feature of all nutritional surveys since their ultimate objective is to assess levels of health of individuals or of population groups in relation to food they consume. There are a number of physical signs, some specific and many non-specific, known to be associated with states of malnutrition. However clinical signs have the following drawbacks:—

(a) Malnutrition cannot be quantified on the basis of clinical signs.
(b) Many deficiencies are unaccompanied by physical signs.
(c) Lack of specificity and subjective nature of most of the physical signs.

2. *Anthropometry:* Anthropometric measurements such as height, weight, skin fold thickness and arm circumference are valuable indications of nutritional status. If anthropometric measurements are recorded over a period of time, they reflect the

patterns of growth and development and how individuals deviate from the average at various ages in body size, build and nutritional status.

3. *Biochemical assessment:—*

(a) Laboratory tests:—

  (i) Hb estimation: It is an important laboratory test that is carried out in nutritional surveys.

  (ii) Stool and urine: Stool should be examined for intestinal parasites. Urine should examined for albumin and sugar.

(b) Biochemical tests: With increasing knowledge of the metabolic functions of vitamins and minerals, assessment of nutritional status by clinical signs has given way to more precise biochemical tests.

Some biochemical tests in nutritional surveys are:—

Nutrient	Method	Normal value
Vit. A	Serum retinol	20 mcg/dl
Thiamine	Thiamine pyrophosphate (TPP) stimulation of RBC transketolase activity.	1.00-1.23 (ratio)
Riboflavin	RBC glutathione reductase activity stimulated by FAD	1.0-1.2 (ratio)
Niacin	Urine N-methyl nicotinamide	(not reliable)
	Serum folate	6.0 mcg/ml
	Red cell folate	160 mcg/ml

Vit. B_{12}	Serum Vit. B_{12} concentration	160 mg/l
Vit. C	Leucocyte ascorbic acid	15mcg/10^8cells
Vit. K	Prothrombin time	11-16 seconds

Biochemical tests are expensive and time consuming so they are usually applied in a sub-population.

4. *Functional indicators:* Functional indices of nutritional status are emerging as an important class of diagnostic tools. Some of the functional indicators are given in the table below:—

System	Nutrients
1. Structural integrity	
Erythrocyte fragility	Vit. E, Se
Capillary fragility	Vit. C
Tensile strength	Cu
2. Host defense	
Leucocyte chemotaxis	P/E, Zn
Leucocyte phagocytic capacity	P/E, Fe
Leucocyte bactericidal capacity	P/E, Fe, Se
T cell blastogenesis	P/E, Zn
Delayed cutaneous hypersensitivity	P/E, Zn
3. Hemostasis	
Prothrombin time	Vit. K
4. Reproduction	
Sperm count	Energy, Zn
5. Nerve function	
Nerve conduction	P/E, Vit. B, Vit. B_{12}
Dark adaptation	Vit. A, Zn

EEG	P/E
6. **Work capacity**	
Heart rate	P/E, Fe
Vasopressor response	Vit. C

5. *Assessment of dietary intake:—*

A dietary survey may be carried out by one of the following methods:—

(i) Weighing of raw foods: The survey team visits the house-hold and weighs all food that is going to be cooked and eaten as well as that which is wasted or discarded. The duration may vary from 1 to 21 days but commonly 7 days which is called one dietary cycle.

(ii) Weighing of cooked food.

(iii) Oral questionaire method: Inquiries are made retrospectively about the nature and quantity of foods eaten during the previous 24 to 48 hours.

The data collected has to be transformed into:—

(a) Mean intake of food in terms are cereals, pulses, vegetables, fruits, milk, meat, fish and eggs.

(b) The mean intake of nutrients per adult man value or consumption unit.

6. *Vital statistics:* An analysis of vital statistics – mortality and morbidity data – will identify groups at high risk and indicate the extent of risk to community.

7. *Assessment of ecological factors:* A study of ecological factors comprises the following:—

(i) Food balance sheets: In this supplies are related to census population to derive levels of food consumption in terms of per capita supply availability.

(b) Socio-economic factors: Are like family size, occupation, income, education, customs, cultural patterns in relation to feeding practices of children.

(c) Health and educational services: PHC services, feeding and immunization programmes should also be taken into consideration.

(d) Conditioning influences: These include parasitic, bacterial and viral infections which precipitate malnutrition.

Health status of under-five children can be assessed by the following methods:—

1. *Weight:* Infants born to well-fed mothers in India weigh about 3.2 kg at birth.

    Baby doubles its birth weight by 5 months of age, trebles it by 1 year. By the end of 2nd year birth weight gets quadrupled.

2. *Height:* In first year of life, the body lengths by about 50%. In the second year another 12 to 13 cms are added. After that growth is 5-6 cms every year.

3. *Head and chest circumference:* At birth, the head circumference is larger than the chest circumference.

4. *Growth chart:* It is the visible display of the child's physical growth and development, child should be weighed atleast once every month during the first year.

Every 2 month during second year, and every 3 month thereafter till 5 to 6 years of age. When the child's weight is plotted on the growth chart at monthly intervals against his or her age, it gives *weight-for-age* growth curve.

MILESTONES OF DEVELOPMENT

	Motor Development	Language development	Adaptive development	Socio-personal development
6-8 weeks				Looks at mother & smiles.
3 months	Holds head erect.			
4-5 months		Listening.	Begins to reach out for objects.	Recognizes mother.
6-8 months	Sits without support.	Experimenting with noise.	Transfers objects hand to hand.	Enjoys hide and seek.
9-10 months	Crawling.	Increasing range of sounds.	Releases objects.	Suspicious of strangers.
10-11 months	Stands with support.	First words.		
12-14 months	Walks with wide base.		Builds.	
18-21 months	Walks with narrow base; beginning to run.	Joining words together.	Beginning to explore.	
2 years	Runs.	Short sentences		Day by day.

Q.6 Write short notes on:—

(i) **Standard deviation.**

(ii) **Vitamin A prophylaxis.**

(iii) **Presumptive treatment of malaria.**

(iv) **Iodized salt.**

(v) **Perinatal mortality rate.**

(vi) **Mental retardation.**

Ans. (i) Standard deviation: The standard deviation is the most frequently used measure of deviation. In simple terms, it is defined as "Root – Means – Square – Deviation". The standard deviation is calculated from basic formula:—

$$SD = \sqrt{\frac{\Sigma(x-\bar{x})^2}{\eta}}$$

When the sample size is more than 30, the above basic formula may be used without modification. For smaller samples, the above formula tends to underestimate the standard deviation and therefore needs correction, which is done by substituting the denominator ($\eta-1$) for η.

Modified formula is:—

$$SD = \sqrt{\frac{\Sigma(x-\bar{x})^2}{\eta-1}}$$

Basic significance of S D is that it is an abstract number, that it gives us an idea of the 'spread' of the dispersion; that the larger the S D, the greater the dispersion of values about the mean.

(ii) Vitamin A prophylaxis: National programme for control of blindness is to administer a single massive dose of an oily preparation of Vitamin A containing 200,000 IU orally to all preschool children in the community every 6 months through peripheral health workers. This programme was launched by the Ministry of Health and Family Welfare in 1970. The basis of the technology was developed at the National Institute of Nutrition in Hyderabad. An evaluation of the programme has revealed a significant reduction in Vitamin A deficiency in children.

(iii) Presumptive treatment of malaria:—

There are two different approaches to malaria control:—

(a) Management of malaria cases.

(b) Active intervention to control or interrupt malaria transmission with community participation.

(a) *Management of malaria cases:—*

1. Case detection:—

(i) Malaria eradication: The objective is to detect and eliminate the human reservoir of infection. The case detection is both active and passive.

Active case detection is based on domiciliary house visits twice a month by paid health workers and collection of blood films from all fever cases or those just recovered from an attack of fever for microscopic diagnosis.

Passive case detection is done by state health agencies such as PHC, subcentre, hospitals and dispensaries.

(ii) Malaria control : Major emphasis is placed on diagnosis of the disease and its treatment at the peripheral level mostly on clinical grounds.

2. Chemotherapy:—

Antimalarial drugs:—

- To prevent deaths.
- To reduce morbidity.

(i) Clinical treatment:—

In the context malaria control, treatment of malaria must be effective, whether it is provided at the health centre immediately after the microscopic diagnosis.

(ii) Radical treatment: This is treatment of confirmed malaria cases so that complete elimination of parasite is achieved, thus preventing a relapse or reoccurrence.

(iii) In highly endemic areas, mass prophylaxis is suggested.

Active intervention measures:—

(i) Stratification of the problem: It is an essential feature for the planning and development of a sound control strategy to maximize the utilization of available resources.
(ii) Vector control strategies

Vector control: Mosquito Control Measures.

1. *Anti-larval measures:—*

(a) Environmental control: Reducing their breeding places. This is known as source reduction and comprises of minor engineering methods such as filling, leveling and drainage of breeding places:—

Culex: Reducing domestic and predomestic sources of breeding such as cesspools and open ditches.

Aedes: Environment should be cleaned up and got rid of water holding containers such as discarded tins, empty pots, broken bottles, etc.

Anopheles: Breeding places should be looked for and abolished by appropriate engineering measures.

Mansonia: Reduce the aquatic plants.

(b) Chemical control: Commonly used larvicides are:—

   (i) Mineral oils.

   (ii) Paris green.

   (iii) Synthetic insecticides.

Mineral oils: The application of oil to water is one of the oldest known mosquito control measures. Since the life cycle of a mosquito occupies about 8 days or so it is customary to apply oil once a week on all breeding places.

Paris green: It is a stomach poison and to be effective it must be ingested by the larvae. Anopheles are surface feeders so it is easily killed by Paris green and for bottom feeders Paris green is applied in granular formation.

Synthetic insecticides: E.g., fenthion, chlorpyrifos and abate are effective larvicides. These organophosphorus compounds hydrolyze quickly in water.

(c) Biological control: A wide range of small fish feed readily on mosquito larvae. The best known are Gambusia offense and Lebister reticulatus.

2. *Anti-adult measures:—*

(a) Residual sprays: E.g., DDT 1-2 grams of pure DDT per sq. metre are applied 3 times a year to walls and other surfaces where mosquitoes rest.

(b) Space sprays: These are those where the insecticidal formulation is sprayed into the atmosphere in the form of mist or fog to kill insects.

Common space sprays are:—

(i) Pyrethrum extract: Pyrethrum flowers form an excellent space sprays.

It has the active principle *pyrethrin* which is a nerve poison and kills the insects instantly on mere contact.

(ii) Residual insecticide: Malathion and jenitrothin.

(c) Genetic control:—

   (i) Sterile male technique.

   (ii) Cytoplasmic incompatibility.

   (iii) Chromosomal translocations.

   (iv) Sex distortion.

   (v) Gene replacement.

3. *Protection against mosquito bites:*—

(a) Mosquito net: It offers protection against mosquito bites during sleep. The net should be white to allow easy detection of mosquitoes. Best pattern is a rectangular net.

The size of opening should not exceed 0.0475 inch in diameter. The number of holes in one square inch are usually 150.

(b) Screening: Of buildings with copper or bronze gauze having 16 meshes to the inch is recommended. The aperture should not be larger than 0.0475 inch.

(c) Repellents: Like Diethyl toluamide is active against fatigans.

(iv) Iodized salt: The iodization of salt is now the most widely used prophylactic public health measure against endemic goitre. In India the level of iodization is fixed under the prevention of Food Adulteration Act (PFA) and is not less than 30 ppm at the production point and not less than 15 ppm of iodine at the consumer level.

Iodized salt is most economical, convenient and effective means of mass prophylaxis in endemic areas. Under the national IDD control activities, the Govt. of India proposed to completely replace common salt with iodized salt in a phased manner by 1992.

(v) Perinatal mortality rate: The term "perinatal mortality" includes both late fetal deaths (still births) and early neonatal deaths.

$$\text{Perinatal mortality rate} = \frac{\text{Late fetal deaths} + \text{Deaths under week} \times 1000}{\text{Live births in a year}}$$

Causes of perinatal mortality: The cause of death are:

(a) Antenatal causes:—

1. Maternal diseases:—

(i) Hypertension

(ii) Cardiovascular diseases

(iii) Diabetes

(iv) Tuberculosis

(v) Anemia

2. Pelvic diseases:—
(i) Uterine myomas
(ii) Endometriosis
(iii) Ovarian tumors

3. Anatomical defects:—
(i) Uterine anomalies
(ii) Incompetent cervix

4. Endocrine imbalance and inadequate uterine preparation.
5. Blood incompatibilities.
6. Malnutrition.
7. Toxemias of pregnancy.
8. Antepartum hemorrhages.
9. Congenital defects.
10. Advanced maternal age.

(b) Intranatal causes:—
(1) Birth injuries.
(2) Asphyxia.
(3) Prolonged effort time.
(4) Obstetric complications.

(c) Postnatal causes:—
1. Prematurity.

2. Respiratory distress syndrome.
3. Infections: Respiratory and alimentary.
4. Congenital anomalies.

(vi) Mental retardation: Mental retardation may be congenital or acquired. Mental retardation is a state when psychological abilities associated with intelligence do not develop to a normal level. A child less than 75 IQ is considered mentally retarded. WHO has classified mental retardation as follows:—

(a) Profound   IQ less than 20
(b) Severe   IQ 20-35
(c) Moderate   IQ 36-51
(d) Mild   IQ 52-67

Factors affecting mental retardation in children are:—

(a) Genetic.
(b) Defective hearing.
(c) Nutritional deficiencies.
(d) Psychological deprivation during first five years of life.
(e) Birth injuries.

Q.7 Write briefly aims, objective and strategies of National Family Welfare Programme.

Ans. Aim: The aim of National Family Welfare Programme is to control the population by family planning measures.

Objective: Government of India launched the National Family Planning Programme in 1952. The programme is exploratory in nature along with the distribution of contraceptives through the clinics.

Strategies:—

1. In order to make it a practical success, the programme has been integrated with other health services.
2. Original base is made at subcenter, which are in turn supervised by PHC, district hospitals at state and central levels. In addition, there are family welfare centers, hospitals, dispensaries, mobile sterilization, IUCD units and voluntary agencies, which are conducting family welfare programmes.
3. Integration of family planning programme with maternity and child health services; increased motivation for post-delivery sterilization, more facilities for abortion under liberalised abortion law.
4. There is direct correlation between illiteracy and fertility. It is therefore suggested to lay more stress and give higher priority especially to the aspect of a girl's education.
5. There should be more stress on child healthcare, so as to encourage more survival of children.
6. Breast feeding should be encouraged.
7. Raising the age of marriage for both boys and girls is also expected to yield better results.
8. Our basic enemy is poverty to encounter which a *Minimum Needs Programme* was announced for the fifth five year plan. Fertility rate is directly proportional to the per capita income of people.

9. Since monetary incentives have been helpful in the promotion of family planning especially among the poorer classes, it is proposed to retain this incentive.

10. Training and research programmes with regard to the reproductive biology and contraception is also intensified at the five central and 47 regional training centers in the country.

11. Multi-media motivation strategy through radio, T.V., press, cinemas and audiovisual aids.

12. Motivation of the people in the reproductive age group to accept the family planning programme is the important aim.

Q.8 What are the common nutritional problems in India? Discuss the preventive and control measures.

Ans. Common nutritional problems in India are:—

1. Low birth weight.

2. Protein energy malnutrition.

3. Xerophthalmia.

4. Nutritional anemia.

5. Iodine deficiency disorders.

6. Endemic fluorosis.

7. Lathyrism.

Prevention and control measures are:—

1. *Low birth weight:—*

(a) Direct interventions:—

   (i) Increasing food intake: Pregnant mother's diet should be increased. Direct intervention covers supplementary feeding, distribution of iron and folic acid tablets, fortification and enrichment of foods, etc.

   (ii) Controlling infections: Maternal infections should be diagnosed and treated or otherwise prevented.

   (iii) Early detection and treatment of medical disorders: Include hypertension, toxemias and diabetes.

(b) Indirect interventions:—

   (i) Family planning.

   (ii) Prenatal advice: Avoidance of heavy work load and smoking during pregnancy.

   (iii) Improvements in socio-economic conditions.

2. *Protein calorie malnutrition:* It is a major health problem in India. It occurs particularly in weaklings and children in the first years of life. It is not only an important cause of childhood mortality and morbidity, but also leads to permanent impairment of physical and possibly of mental growth.

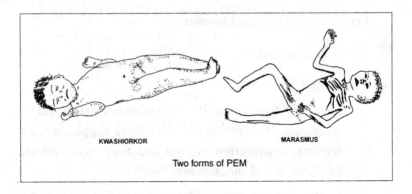
Two forms of PEM

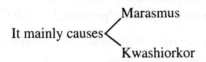

It mainly causes { Marasmus, Kwashiorkor }

Causes:—

(a) Inadequate intake of food, both in quantity and quality.//
(b) Infections notably diarrhea, respiratory infections, measles, intestinal worms.//
(c) Poor environmental conditions.//
(d) Large family.//
(e) Poor maternal health.//
(f) Failure of lactation.//
(g) Premature termination of breast feeding.

The first indication of PCM is *being underweight for age.*

Preventive measures are:—

Health promotion:—

1. Measures directed to pregnant and lactating mothers.

2. Promotion of breast feeding.
3. Development of low-cost weaning foods.
4. Measures to improve family diet.
5. Nutritional education – promotion of correct feeding practices.
6. Health economics.
7. Family planning.

Specific protections:—

1. Child's diet must contain protein and energy rich foods.
2. Immunization.
3. Food fortification.

Early diagnosis and treatment:—

1. Periodic surveillance.
2. Early diagnosis of lag in growth.
3. Early diagnosis and treatment of infections and diarrhea.
4. Development of programmes for early rehydration of children with diarrhea.

Rehabilitation:—

1. Nutritional rehabilitation services.
2. Hospital treatment.
3. Follow up care.

3. Xerophthalmia:—

(a) Short term action: Administration of a large dose of vitamin A orally to all vulnerable groups on periodic basis.

(b) Medium term action: It is fortification of foods with vitamin A. Addition of vitamin A to dalda, sugar, salt, tea, etc.

(c) Long term action: Reduction or elimination of factors contributing to ocular diseases.

> (i) Persuading people in general and mothers in particular, to consume dark green leafy vegetables.
>
> (ii) Promotion of breast feeding.
>
> (iii) Improvements in environmental health as ensuring safe and adequate water supply and construction and maintenance of pit latrines.
>
> (iv) Immunization against infectious diseases such as measles.
>
> (v) Better feeding of infants and young children.
>
> (vi) Improved health services for mothers and children.
>
> (vii) Social health education.

4. *Nutritional anemia:—*

(a) Iron and folic acid supplementation.
Dosage:—

(i) Mothers: One tablet of iron and folic acid containing 60 mg of elemental iron and 0.5 mg of folic acid. Daily administration continued until 2 to 3 months after Hb has returned to normal.

(ii) Children: Screening test for anemia may be done in infants at 6 months, 1 year and 2 years of age. One tablet of iron and folic acid containing 20 mg of elemental iron and 0.1 mg of folic acid.

(b) Iron fortification: Ferric orthophosphate or ferrous sulphate with sodium bisulfate was enough to fortify salt with iron.

(c) Others strategies include changing dietary habits, control of parasites and nutritional education.

5. *Iodine deficiency disorders:—*

Four essential components of National Goitre Control:—

(i) Iodized salt: It is used as a prophylactic measures against goiter; level of iodization is not less than 30 ppm at production point and not less than 15 ppm of iodine at consumer level.

(ii) Iodized oil: Intramuscular injection of iodized oil. Advantage is that an average dose of 1 ml will provide protection for about 4 years.

(iii) Iodine monitoring:—

    (a) Iodine excretion determination.

    (b) Determination of iodine in water, soil and food as a part of epidemiological studies.

    (c) Determination of iodine in salt for quality control.

(iv) Manpower training: It is vital for the success of control that health workers and others engaged in the programme be fully trained in all aspects of goitre control.

(v) Mass communication: It is a powerful tool for nutritional education. It should be fully used in goitre control work.

6. *Endemic Fluorosis:—*

(a) Changing the water source: One solution to the problem is to find a new source of drinking water with lower fluoride content.

(b) *Chemical treatment:* Water can be chemically defluoridated. It involves the addition of two chemicals (viz. lime and alum) in sequence followed by flocculation, sedimentation and filtration.

7. Lathyrism:—

The possible preventive and control measures are:—

(a) Vitamin C prophylaxis: By daily administration of 500-1000 mg of ascorbic acid for a week or so the damages could be repaired.

(b) Banning the crop.

(c) Removal of the toxin:—

   (i) Steeping method: Since toxins are water soluble, they can be removed by soaking the pulse in hot water. A large quantity of water is boiled and pulse is soaked in hot water for 2 hours, after which the soaked water is drained off completely. The pulse washed again with clean water, then drained off and dried in the sun.

   (ii) Parboiling: Simple soaking in lime water overnight followed by boiling is credited to destroy the toxin.

(d) Education: Public must be educated on the dangers of consuming Khesari dal.

(e) Genetic approach: Certain strains of lathyrus contain very low levels of toxin (0.1%), so these strains must be cultivated.

Q.9 Write short notes on:—

(i) Oral rehydration therapy.

(ii) Fertility indicators.

(iii) **Differenciate – Infection, infestation and contamination.**

(iv) **Health problems of school children.**

(v) **Endemic, epidemic and pandemic.**

Ans. (i) Oral rehydration therapy:—

The aim of ORT is to prevent dehydration and reduce mortality.

Packets of "Oral Rehydration Mixture" are now freely available at the PHC, sub-centers and hospitals. The contents of the packet are to be dissolved in one litre of drinking water. The solution should be made fresh daily and used within 24 hours. A simple mixture consisting of table salt (5g) and sugar (20 g) dissolved in 1 litre of drinking water may be safely used until a proper mixture is obtained.

The actual amount given will depend on the patient's desire to drink and by surveillance of signs of dehydration.

Older children and adults should be given as much as they want, in addition to ORS solution.

Mothers should be taught how to administer ORS solution to their children.

(a) For children under 2 years of age give a teaspoon every 1 to 2 minutes or offer frequent sips out of a cup, for older children. Adults may drink as much as they like.

(b) If the child vomits, wait for 10 minutes, then try again, giving the solution slowly, a spoonful every 2 to 3 minutes.

(c) If the child wants to drink more ORS solution than the estimated amount and does not vomit, there can be no harm in feeding him/her more.

(d) If the child is breast fed, nursing should be pursued during treatment with ORS solution.

(e) Non-breast fed infants under 6 months age should be given an additional 100-200 ml of clean water during the first four hours.

(ii) Fertility indicators:—

There are a number of fertility indicators given below:--

1. *Birth rate:* The number of live births per 1000 estimated mid-year population in a given year.

$$\text{Birth rate} = \frac{\text{Number of live births during the year}}{\text{Estimated mid-year population}} \times 1000$$

2. *General fertility rate:* "Number of live births per 1000 women in the reproductive age group in a given year".

$$\text{GFR} = \frac{\text{Number of live births in an area during the year}}{\text{Mid-year female population age 15-44 in the same area in same year.}} \times 1000$$

3. General marital fertility rate (GMFR): It is the number of live births per 1000 married women in the reproductive age group in a given year.

4. *Age specific fertility rate:* "Number of live births in a year to 1000 women in any specified age group".

5. *Age specific marital fertility rate:* It is the number of live births in a year to 1000 married women in any specified age group.

6. *Total fertility Rate:* Total fertility rate represents the average number of children a women would have if she were to pass through her reproductive years bearing children at the same rate as the women now in each age group.

7. *Total marital fertility rate:* Average number of children that

would be born to a married woman if she experience the current fertility pattern through-out her reproductive span.

8. *Gross reproductive rate (GRR)*: Average number of girls that would be born to a woman if she experiences the current fertility pattern throughout her reproductive span.

9. Net reproduction rate (NRR): NRR is defined as the number of daughters a newborn girl will bear during her life time assuming fixed age specific fertility and mortality rates.

10. *Child-woman ratio*: It is the number of children 0-4 years age per 1000 women of child bearing age usually defined as 15-44 or 49 years of age.

11. *Pregnancy ratio*: It is the ratio of number of pregnancies in a year to married women in the ages 15-44 years.

12. *Abortion rate*: The number of all types of abortion usually per 1000 women of child bearing age.

13. *Abortion ratio:* Number of abortions performed

$$\frac{\text{in a given period}}{\substack{\text{Number of live births} \\ \text{in the same period}}}$$

14. *Marriage rate*: It is the number of marriages in the year per 1000 population.

$$\text{Crude marriage rate} = \frac{\text{Number of marriages in the year} \times 1000}{\text{Mid-year population}}$$

(iii) Infection, infestation and contamination:—

Infection: The entry and development or multiplication of an infectious agent in the body of man and animal. It also implies that the body responds in some way to defend itself against the invader either in the form of a immune response or disease. An infection does not always cause illness.

There are several levels of infection; colonization, sub-clinical or inapparent infection latent infection and clinical infection.

Infestation: For men or animals the lodgement, development and reproduction of arthropods on the surface of the body or in the clothing eg., lice, itch mite.

Contamination: The presence of an infectious agent on the body surface; also on or in clothes, beddings, toys, surgical instruments or dressings or others substances including water, milk and food.

(iv) Health problems of school children:—

The main health problems of school children are:—

(a) Malnutrition.

(b) Infectious diseases.

(c) Intestinal parasites.

(d) Diseases of skin, eye and ear.

(e) Dental caries.

(a) *Malnutrition*: To prevent malnutrition among children mid day meal is given:—

(i) Meal should be a supplement not a substitute.

(ii) Meal should provide 1/3rd energy, 1/2 proteins.

(iii) Cost of meal should be low.

(iv) Should be prepared in the school.

(v) Locally available food should be used.

(vi) Menu should be changed.

(b) *Infectious diseases*: Communicable disease control through immunization. A record of all immunizations should be maintained as a part of school health services.

(c) *Intestinal parasites*: Pure water should be provided to students, regular clinical examination of the child is necessary, stool examination, growth monitoring should be periodically done.

(d) *Eye health services*: Schools should be responsible for early detection of refractive errors, treatment of squint, amblyopia and detection and treatment of eye infections such as trachoma. Administration of vitamin A to children.

(e) *Dental health*: Regular dental examination. There should be inspection of teeth, cleaning which prevent gum troubles. Dental hygiene should be taught to children.

(v) **Endemic, epidemic and pandemic:—**

Ans. *Endemic:* It refers to the constant presence of a disease or infections agent within a given geographic area or population group without importation from outside, eg., common cold.

An endemic disease when conditions are favorable may burst into an epidemic.

Epidemic: An unusual occurrance of disease in excess of expected frequency is called epidemic. Amount of disease occurring in the past in the absence of an epidemic defines the "expected frequency".

Eg., epidemic of measles, chickenpox and slow epidemic of non-communicable diseases like CHD, hypertension.

Pandemic: An epidemic usually affecting a large proportion of the population occurring over a wide geographic area such as a section of a nation, entire nation, continent or the world.

II B.H.M.S. 1998

PART A

Q.1 What do you understand by rehabilitation in disease control? Describe its role in any national programme.

Ans. Rehabilitation is defined as "the combined and coordinated use of medical, social, educational and vocational measures for training, retraining the individual to the highest possible level of functional ability". It includes all measures aimed at reducing the impact of disabling and handicapping conditions and at enabling the disabled and handicapped to achieve social integration. Social integration is active participation of disabled and handicapped people in the main stream of community life.

The following areas of concern in rehabilitation have been identified:—

(a) Medical rehabilitation: Restoration of function.

(b) Vocational rehabilitation: Restoration of the capacity to earn a livelihood.

(c) Social rehabilitation: Restoration of family and social relationships.

(d) Psychological rehabilitation: Restoration of personal dignity and confidence.

The aim of rehabilitation is to make productive people out of non-productive people.

Role of rehabilitation in leprosy control:—

Leprosy patients develop physical disabilities eg., drop foot, claw toes, hammer toes, plantar ulcers, etc.

Rehabilitation is, therefore, an integral part of leprosy control. It must begin as soon as the disease is diagnosed. The cheapest and surest rehabilitation is to prevent physical deformities and adequate treatment. The measures taken in this direction are called "preventive rehabilitation".

Rehabilitation measures may appear to be simple. They require planned and systemic actions – medical, surgical, social, educational and counseling and health education for training or retraining of the individual to the highest possible level of functional ability.

Q.2 What dietary advice will you give to:—

(a) A diabetic patient

(b) A hypertensive patient.

(c) A rheumatic mother during pregnancy.

(d) An asthmatic patient.

Ans. (a) A diabetic patient:—

He has to:—

(i) Maintain blood glucose as close within normal limits.

(ii) To maintain ideal body weight.

Diet: Small balanced meals more frequently.

The main nutrients in terms of proteins, fats and carbohydrates are given below:—

Proteins: Should be 1-1.5gm/kg of body weight. Content should be reduced in case of high blood urea.

Fats: Should provide 25-35% of total calories and should be mostly unsaturated.

Carbohydrates: Should not be less than 100 gms daily in older to prevent ketosis. Usually a supply of less than 15% carbohydrates may lead to ketosis. In general, carbohydrates should form 50-60% of the total calories and should be wholesome rather than being refined.

(b) A hypertensive patient:—

Following dietary changes should be followed:—

(i) Reduction of fat intake to 20-30% of total energy intake.

(ii) Consumption of saturated fats must be limited to less than 10% of total energy intake; some of the reduction in saturated fat may be made up by mono and poly-unsaturated fats.

(iii) A reduction of dietary cholesterol to below 100 mg per 1000 kcal per day.

(iv) An increase in complex carbohydrate consumption.

(v) Avoidance of alcohol consumption; reduction of salt intake to 5 g daily or less.

(c) A rheumatic mother during pregnancy:—

The patient should abstain from taking cold food. The food

should be taken hot or worm. Also, things like curd, potato, brinjal, rice, beans, etc. should not be taken.

(d) An asthmatic patient: An asthmatic patient should not be given the food items which precipitate the attack.

Eg., cream, curd, etc.

A balanced diet should be given to the patient but cold things should not be given. Always try to give them seasonal food.

Q.3 What is air pollution? Describe in detail its control measures.

Ans. When there is excessive concentration of a foreign matter in the outdoor atmosphere which is harmful to man, it is called air pollution.

For control measures—

Methods taken by the government to control air pollution are:—

1. *Containment:* Prevention of escape of toxic substances into the ambient air. Containment can be achieved by a variety of engineering methods such as enclosure, ventilation and air cleaning.

2. *Replacement:* This is replacing a technological process causing air pollution by a new process that does not cause any pollution.

3. *Dilution:* Is valid so long as it is within the self leaning capacity of the environment. The establishment of "green belts" between industrial and residential areas is an attempt at dilution.

4. *Legislation:* Many countries have adopted legislation for control of air pollution.

5. *International action:* To deal with air pollution on a world wide scale, the WHO has established an international network of laboratories for the monitoring and study of air pollution.

The Govt. is converting the diesel buses into CNG which is environment friendly. Aslo, Metro Rail Project is being completed at a very high speed, which will decongest the roads and make the air of Delhi more clean. Also, all the pollution causing factories have been shifted out of Delhi. Many flyovers have been built so that the vehicles spend less time on red lights which causes pollution.

PART B

Q.4 What preventive and control measure will you advice for hookworm problem in a community/

Ans. Diseases transmitted by indiscriminate defection are:—

(a) Typhoid fever.
(b) Paratyphoid fever.
(c) Dysenteries.
(d) Diarrhea.
(e) Cholera.
(g) Hookworms.
(h) Ascariasis.
(i) Infective hepatitis.
(j) Prevention and control of hookworm

Prevention and control involves four approaches:—

1. Sanitary disposal of feces.
2. Chemotherapy.
3. Correction of anemia.
4. Health education.

1. *Sanitary technology*: Long term solution of the problem is the sanitary disposal of human excreta through the installation of sewage disposal system in urban areas. This alone will prevent soil pollution.

2. *Chemotherapy*: Periodic case finding and treatment of all infected persons in the community will reduce the worm burden and frequency of transmission.

3. *Treatment of anemia*: When anemia is severe it should be treated. A cheap and effective treatment is ferrous sulphate 200 mg, three time a day, orally and continued upto 3 months after the Hb has risen to 12 g/100ml.

4. *Health education:* Community involvement through health education is an important aspect in the control of hookworm infection. Health education should be aimed at the use of sanitary latrines and prevention of soil pollution.

Q.5 Discuss health education in school for:—

(a) Prevention of drug addiction:

(b) Sex education at school age.

Ans. (a) Health education is an important element of school health programme. The teachers give health education to children.

To prevent today's student from becoming tomorrow's drug addicts, it is necessary to warn them in the childhood about the diseases associated with drug addiction. Eg., cigarette smoking is a public health problem that should be talked in schools. The teachers should pay attention toward students to prevent the origin of poor health habits in them. Posters and charts showing the diseases and dread associated with addiction should be pasted in schools.

(b) Sex education at school age: Children should be given sex education at school age by their teachers and their course should also include the sex education because of so many sexually transmitted diseases like AIDS, Syphilis, etc., Due to lack of knowledge, the students are curious towards sex and they want to experiment with it. This way they ruin there life by causing harm to their health and their careers and by the time they realize their mistakes, it is too late. Later they are guilty conscious. To prevent children from the hazards of lack of knowledge, the teachers should give them sex education so that they get familiar with it and no curiosity is left in them. They should also be taught about STD.

Q.6 Discuss the epidemiology & control of malaria in India?

Ans. Epidemiology of malaria:—

Agent factors: Malaria in man is caused by:—

    (a) P. vivax.

    (b) P. falciparum.

    (c) P. malariae.

    (d) P. ovale.

Plasmodium vivax has widest geographical distribution.

Life history: Malarial parasite has 2 cycles:—

    (a) Human   (b) Mosquito
       cycle   cycle

Human cycle: Caesural cycle begins when the mosquito bites and injects sporozoites.

There are 3 phases:—

(a) Hepatic phase: The sporozoites disappear within 60 minutes from peripheral circulation. Some are destroyed, others reach the live cell. The number of merozoites produced from a sporozoite differ in each species.

(b) Erythrocyte phase: Many of the merozoites are quickly destroyed but a significant number attack RBCs. The merozoites then penetrate RBCs and pass through stages of trophozoite and schizont. The erythrocytic phase ends with liberation of merozoites which further infect fresh RBCs.

(c) Gametogeny: Some erythrocytic forms do not divide but become male and female gametocytes.

Mosquito cycle: (Sexual cycle): When gametocytes are ingested by vector sexual cycle begins.

Host factors:—

(a) Age: Malaria affects all ages.

(b) Sex: Males are more frequently exposed.

(c) Race: Sickle cell trait have milder illness.

(d) Pregnancy: Increases risk of malaria.

(e) Socio-economic development: Malaria has disappeared from developed countries.

(f) Housing: Ill ventilated and ill lighted houses provide ideal indoor resting places for mosquitos.

(g) Population mobility: People migrating from one region to another may carry the malarial parasite with them.

(h) Occupation: Malaria is predominant in agriculture practices.

(i) Human habits: Habit of sleeping outdoors, refusal to accept spraying of houses increases the risk of malaria.

(j) Immunity: It is acquired only after repeated exposure.

Environmental factor:—

(a) Season: Maximum prevalence is from July to November.

(b) Temperature: Optimum temperature between 20° to 30° C.

(c) Humidity: 60% necessary for mosquito survival.

(d) Rainfall: Rain provides more opportunity for breeding of mosquitoes.

Mosquito control measures:—

1. *Anti-larval measures:—*

(a) Environmental control: Reducing their breeding places. This is known as source reduction and comprises of minor engineering methods such as filling, leveling and drainage of breeding places:—

Culex: Reducing domestic and predomestic sources of breeding such as cesspools and open ditches.

Aedes: Environment should be cleaned up and got rid of water holding containers such as discarded tins, empty pots, broken bottles, etc.

Anopheles: Breeding places should be looked for and abolished by appropriate engineering measures.

Mansonia: Reduce the aquatic plants.

(b) Chemical control: Commonly used larvicides are:—

    (i) Mineral oils.

    (ii) Paris green.

    (iii) Synthetic insecticides.

Mineral oils: The application of oil to water is one of the oldest known mosquito control measures. Since the life cycle of a mosquito occupies about 8 days or so it is customary to apply oil once a week on all breeding places.

Paris green: It is a stomach poison and to be effective it must be ingested by the larvae. Anopheles are surface feeders so it is easily killed by Paris green and for bottom feeders Paris green is applied in granular formation.

Synthetic insecticides: E.g., fenthion, chlorpyrifos and abate are effective larvicides. These organophosphorus compounds hydrolyze quickly in water.

(c) Biological control: A wide range of small fish feed readily on mosquito larvae. The best known are Gambusia offense and **Lebister reticulatus**.

2. *Anti-adult measures:*—

    (a) Residual sprays: E.g., DDT 1-2 grams of pure DDT per sq.

metre are applied 3 times a year to walls and other surfaces where mosquitoes rest.

(b) Space sprays: These are those where the insecticidal formulation is sprayed into the atmosphere in the form of mist or fog to kill insects.

Common space sprays are:—

(i) Pyrethrum extract: Pyrethrum flowers form an excellent space sprays.

It has the active principle *pyrethrin* which is a nerve poison and kills the insects instantly on mere contact.

(ii) Residual insecticide: Malathion and jenitrothin.

(c) Genetic control:—

    (i) Sterile male technique.

    (ii) Cytoplasmic incompatibility.

    (iii) Chromosomal translocations.

    (iv) Sex distortion.

    (v) Gene replacement.

3. *Protection against mosquito bites:—*

(a) Mosquito net: It offers protection against mosquito bites during sleep. The net should be white to allow easy detection of mosquitoes. Best pattern is a rectangular net.

The size of opening should not exceed 0.0475 inch in diameter. The number of holes in one square inch are usually 150.

(b) Screening: Of buildings with copper or bronze gauze having

16 meshes to the inch is recommended. The aperture should not be larger than 0.0475 inch.

(c) *Repellents:* Like Diethyl toluamide is active against fatigans.

PART C

Q.7 Describe the functions of district tuberculosis center in the National Tuberculosis Programme in India.

Ans. The National Tuberculosis Programme: It has been in operation since 1962. The goal of NTP is to reduce the problem of tuberculosis in the community sufficiently quickly to the level where it ceases to be a public health problem.

District Tuberculosis Programme (DTP) is the backbone of NTP. The District Tuberculosis Centre (DTC) is the nucleus to DTP. The function of the DTC is to plan, organize and implement the DTP in the entire district in association with general health services.

Their activities include:—

(a) *Case finding:* Sputum examination is done to detect new T.B. cases in rural population. To further improve case finding male health workers are required to collect and fix sputum of the symptomatic cases on the slide during their routine visits to the villages and send the slides to the nearest health center for microscopic examination.

(b) *Treatment:* It is free and is offered on domiciliary basis from all the health institutions. It is organized in such a manner that patients are expected to collect drugs once a month on fixed dates from the nearest treatment centre. When the patient fails to collect his/her drugs on the "due date", a letter is written to him/her and in the event of no response for 7 days a home visit is paid by the hospital staff.

(c) *BCG vaccination:* By UIP, the coverage of BCG has gone up.

(d) *Recording and reporting:* The names and addresses of all the sputum the cases are sent to DTC every Saturday. The DTC registers all sputum positive cases.

(e) *Supervision:* The DTC team visits the peripheral health institutions regularly and helps them in planning and rendering T.B. control services.

The DTC team includes:—

1 District tuberculosis officer.

1 Laboratory technician.

1 Treatment organiser.

1 X-ray technician

1 Non-medical team leader.

1 Statistical assistant.

Prevention and control of T. B.:—

1. It should be a compulsorily notifiable disease.
2. All the sputum positive patients should be isolated till they are sputum negative.

3. All detected cases should be promptly treated with a proper follow up to ensure the continuity of their treatment.
4. Chemoprophylaxis of all known contacts should be undertaken.
5. Early diagnosis and detection of cases.
6. Rehabilitation of the treated cases.
7. Health education of the public so that they should endeavour to avoid exposure to infection and cooperate in BCG vaccination and chemoprophylaxis, etc.
8. Some of the practical methods under the mass screening programme are as follows:—

(i) Mass tuberculin testing is useful in establishing index of infection in a given community.

(ii) Sputum examination for AFB. This is one of the easiest and fruitful methods to uncover many undetected tubercular cases.

(iii) BCG vaccination should be given to new borns below four weeks and the other susceptible individuals to protect against the infection.

Q.8 Discuss in detail consumption of tobacco and its effect on health.

Ans. Tobacco chewing and tobacco smoking causes:—

1. Oral cancer.

2. Lung cancer.

3. Coronary heart disease.

4. Hypertension.

1. *Oral cancer:* Occurs among those who smoked or chewed tobacco. Oral cancer is preceded by some type of pre-cancerous lesion. Cancer almost always occurrs on that side of mouth where the tobacco quid is kept. Pre-cancerous stage precedes the development of cancer.

2. *Lung Cancer:* Tobacco smoking is the main cause of lung cancer. There is a relationship between cigarette smoking and lung cancer. The risk is strongly related to:—

(a) The number of cigarettes smoked.

(b) The age of starting to smoke.

(c) Smoking habits.

(d) Puffs, the nicotine and tar content.

(e) Length of cigarettes.

Those who are highly exposed to "passive smoking" are at increased risk of developing lung cancer. The most noxious component of tobacco smoke are tar, carbon monoxide and nicotine. The carcinogenic is tar. Nicotine and CO, particularly contribute to increased risk.

3. *Coronary heart disease:* Is associated with smoking tobacco because it contains carbon monoxide which induces atherogenesis; nicotine stimulation of adrenergic drive raises both B.P. and myocardial oxygen demand; lipid metabolism with fall in "protective" high-density lipoproteins, etc.

4. *Hypertension:* Smoking, tobacco chewing may contribute to hypertension.

Q.9 Discuss the sanitary conditions of:—

(a) **Five star hotels;**

(b) **Dhabas;**

(c) **Halwai shops;**

(d) **Households.**

Ans. (a) Five star hotels: If the hotel is situated away from filth, open drains, stable, manure pits, etc. it is very good according to sanitation and hygiene aspect. The food which is cooked in hotels is not fresh but it is not reached by flies. Ventilation is there in the rooms. Rooms are very clean. However food sanitation also depend on personal hygiene and habits of food handlers. The handlers should wash their hand every time they serve. Also the sanctation and hygiene of utensils in which food is served is improtant.

(b) Dhabas: These are usually situated near some open drain. There is no ventilation. The utensils are not clean. The food handlers are not cleanly dressed. Flies suround the food and the rooms are not very clean. A dhaba is usually very congested. Hence, the food served in dhaba is not good according to sanitation and hygiene.

(c) Halwai shops: These are always reached by flies. These flies contaminate the food. Rats live in these shops and contaminate the food. Food is not fresh. Rooms are not clean. There is no ventilation. The utensils are not clean. Food handlers are not educated and they don't know anything about personal hygiene. So food served in a halwai shop is also bad according to sanitation and hygiene.

(d) Households: At home, food is good according to sanitation and hygiene because fresh vegetables which are washed properly are used. The food is never touched by flies. Home is a clean place to eat the food. The personal hygiene maintained is very good for sanitation of food, utensils are also cleaned properly. So, the food which we cook ourself and eat in our home is best according to hygiene and sanitation.

II B.H.M.S. 1999

PART A

Q.1 Describe in detail the natural history of disease giving illustrations.

Ans. Natural history of disease: The term natural history of disease signifies the way in which a disease evolves over time from the earliest stage of its prepathogenesis phase to its termination as recovery, disability or death in the absence of treatment or prevention.

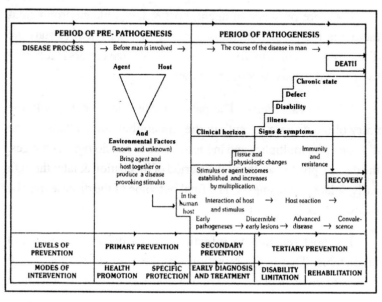

The natural history of disease consists of two phases:—

1. Prepathogenesis phase.
2. Pathogenesis phase.

Prepathogenesis phase: This refers to the period preliminary to the onset of disease in man. The disease agent has not yet entered man; but the factors which favor its interaction with the human host are already existing in the environment.

The causative factors of disease may be classified as:—

(i) Agent.
(ii) Host.
(iii) Environment.

These three factors are referred to as the *epidemiological triad.*

The mere presence of agent, host & favorable environmental factors in the prepathogenesis period is not sufficient to start the disease process in man. *Interaction* of these three factors is required to initiate the disease process in man.

Pathogenesis phase: The pathogenesis phase beings with the entry of the disease "agent" in the susceptible human "host". The disease agent multiplies and induces tissue & physiological changes, the disease progresses through a period of incubation & later through early & late pathogenesis. The final outcome of the disease may be recovery, disability or death.

The host reaction to infection with a disease agent is not predictable. That is the infection may be *clinical* or *subclinical; typical* or *atypical* or the host may become a carrier with or without developing clinical disease as in case of diphtheria & poliomyelitis.

In chronic diseases (e.g., coronary heart disease, hypertension, cancer), the early pathogenesis phase is less dramatic. This phase in chronic disease is referred to as the presymptomatic phase. During this presymptomatic phase there is no manifest disease. The pathological changes are below "clinical horizon". The clinical stage begins when recognizable signs & symptoms appear.

Levels of prevention:—
1. Primary prevention
2. Secondary prevention.
3. Tertiary prevention.

Primary prevention: It can be defined as action taken prior to the onset of disease, which removes the possibility that disease will ever occur. It signifies the intervention in the prepathogenesis phase or a disease or health problem.

Primary prevention may be accomplished by measures designed to promote general health, well-being & quality of life in people or by specific protective measures.

The WHO has recommended the following approaches for primary prevention of chronic diseases:—

(a) Premordial prevention: Prevention of the emergence or development of risk factors in countries or population groups in which they have not yet appealed. For e.g., smoking, eating patterns.

(b) Population (mass) Strategy: It is directed at the whole population irrespective of individual risk factors. For e.g., studies have shown that even a small reduction in the average blood pressure of a population would produce a large reduction in cardiovascular diseases.

(c) High-risk strategy: It aims to bring preventive care to individuals at special risk. This requires detection of individuals at high risk by optimum use of clinical methods.

Secondary prevention: "Action which halts the progress of a disease at its incipient stage & prevents complications".

The specific interventions are:—

(a) Early diagnosis (e.g., screening tests, case finding programmes).
(b) Adequate treatment.

By early diagnosis and adequate treatment, secondary prevention attempts to arrest the disease process, restore health by seeking out unrecognized disease and treating it before reversible pathological changes have taken place.

3. *Tertiary prevention:* It signifies intervention in the late pathogenesis phase. Tertiary prevention can be defined as all measures available to reduce or limit impairments and disabilities. For e.g., treatment even if undertaken late in the natural history of a disease may prevent the sequelae and limit disability.

Modes of intervention:—

(i) Health Promotion.
(ii) Specific Protection.
(iii) Early diagnosis and treatment.
(iv) Disability limitation.
(v) Rehabilitation.

(i) *Health promotion:* It is the process of enabling people to increase control over and to improve health. It is not directed against any particular disease, but is intended to strengthen the host through a variety of approaches (interventions). The well known interventions in this area are:—

(a) Health education.
(b) Environmental modifications.
(c) Nutritional interventions.
(d) Lifestyle and behavioral changes.

(a) Health education: A large number of diseases could be prevented if people are adequately informed about them and if they are encouraged to take necessary precautions in time.

(b) Environmental modifications: Such as provision of safe water; installation of sanitary latrines; control of insects and rodents; improvement of housing, etc.

(c) Nutritional interventions: These comprise of food distribution and nutritional improvement of vulnerable groups, child feeding programmes, food fortifications, nutritional education, etc.

(d) Lifestyle and behavioral changes: The action of prevention in this case is one of individual and community responsibility for health. The physician and each health worker acts as an educator, rather than a therapist.

(ii) *Specific protection:* To avoid disease altogether is the ideal 2but this is possible only in a limited number of cases. The following are some of the currently available interventions aimed at specific protection:—

(a) Immunization.

(b) Use of specific nutrients.

(c) Chemoprophylaxis.

(d) Protection against occupational diseases.

(e) Protection against accidents.

(f) Protection against carcinogens.

(g) Avoidance of allergens.

(h) The control of specific hazards in general environment.

(iii) *Early diagnosis and treatment:* Are main interventions of disease control. The earlier a disease is diagnosed and treated the better it is from the point of view of prognosis and preventing the occurrence of further cases or any longterm disability.

(iv) *Disability limitation:* When a patient reports late in the pathogenesis phase the mode of intervention is disability limitation.

Concept of disability:—

Disease

↓

Impairment

↓

Disability

↓

Handicap

Impairment: Any loss or abnormality of psychological, physiological or anatomical structure or functions.

E.g., loss of foot, defective vision.

Disability: Because of an impairment, the affected person may be unable to carry out certain activities considered normal for his age, sex, etc.

Handicap: It is defined as a disadvantage for a given individual, resulting from an impairment or a disability that limits or prevents the fulfillment of a role that is normal.

(v) *Rehabilitation:* Defined as the combined and coordinated use of medical, social, educational and vocational measures for training and retraining the individual to the highest possible level of functional ability.

Q.2 Discuss the problem of population explosion and its implication on health in our country.

Ans. Population explosion is observed under three readily observable human phenomena:—

(a) Changes in population size.

(b) Composition of the population.

(c) Distribution of population in space.

There are five processes which are continually at work within a population:—

(a) Fertility.

(b) Mortality.

(c) Marriage.

(d) Migration.

(e) Social mobility.

Population in our country is increasing at the rate of 2.1%. India has the second highest population in world.

Population of urban areas has increased due to natural growth and migration from villages because of employment opportunities, attraction of better living conditions and avaibility of social services such as education, health, transport, entertainment, etc. To reduce the population, following measures are applied:—

1. *Age at marriage:* Is increased both for males and females. Females can marry at an age of 18 and above and males at the age of 21 and above.
2. *Duration of married life:* 10 to 25% of births occur within 1-5 years of married life; 50-55% of births within 5-15 years of married life. Births after 25 years of married life are very few.
3. *Spacing of children:* Has a significant impact on the general reduction in fertility eates.
4. *Education:* Especially of girls helps in reduction of population.
5. *Economic status:* The total number of children born declines with an increase in the per capita expenditure of the household.
6. *Caste and religion:* Muslims have a higher fertility rate than Hindus.
7. *Nutrition:* All well-fed societies have low fertility rate.
8. *Family planning:* Is an important factor in fertility reduction.

Health is vitally concerned with population because health in a group depends upon the:—

(i) Dynamic relationship between the number of people.

(ii) The space which they occupy.

(iii) The skill they have acquired in providing for their needs.

Hazards of population explosion are:—

1. *Food production:* It has increased in our country but population increases much faster leading to deficient or less calories per person. If food production doubles in 10 years, the population triples in 10 year.

2. *Clothing:* Against per capita, a minimum of 25 m per annum, the supply is only 14 metres.

3. *Employment* Unemployment is increasing in spite of the creation of additional jobs.

4. *Education front:* We are trying to educate every section of the society, paying special attention to children.

5. *Health programmes:* The increase in population is causing an increase in air, water and soil pollution and general ill health. Our total population ratio stands for 1:5,703 which is still far from the target. Our infant and maternal mortality rate, nutritional status, health of children are affected adversely.

Q.3 Explain briefly:—

(a) **Management of protein energy malnutrition.**

(b) **Criterion for selection of a prize baby in a show.**

(c) **Assesment of the nutrihonal status of a community.**

Ans. (a) Protein calorie malnutrition: It is a major health problem in India. It occurs particularly in weaklings and children in the first years of life. It is not only an important cause of childhood mortality and morbidity, but also leads to permanent impairment of physical and possibly of mental growth.

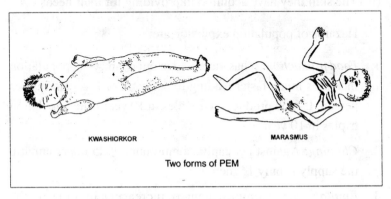

Two forms of PEM

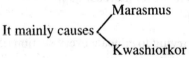

Causes:—

(a) Inadequate intake of food, both in quantity and quality.

(b) Infections notably diarrhea, respiratory infections, measles, intestinal worms.

(c) Poor environmental conditions.

(d) Large family.

(e) Poor maternal health.

(f) Failure of lactation.

(g) Premature termination of breast feeding.

The first indication of PCM is *being underweight for age.*

Preventive measures are:—

Health promotion:—

1. Measures directed to pregnant and lactating mothers.
2. Promotion of breast feeding.
3. Development of low-cost weaning foods.
4. Measures to improve family diet.
5. Nutritional education – promotion of correct feeding practices.
6. Health economics.
7. Family planning.

Specific protections:—

1. Child's diet must contain protein and energy rich foods.
2. Immunization.
3. Food fortification.

Early diagnosis and treatment:—

1. Periodic surveillance.
2. Early diagnosis of lag in growth.
3. Early diagnosis and treatment of infections and diarrhea.
4. Development of programmes for early rehydration of children with diarrhea.

Rehabilitation:—

1. Nutritional rehabilitation services.
2. Hospital treatment.

3. Follow-up care.

(b) Criteria for selection of a prize baby in a baby show, where you are a medical officer on its selection board:—

In a good baby show for selection of a prize baby there are the following things:—

(i) Registration: All infants and babies are to be registered.

(ii) Medical examination: Complete medical examination including height and weight are measured. The child is examined for evidence of disease or defects.

(iii) Parent counseling: About the diet, sleep, test, habits, etc.

(iv) Immunization: Child must be immunized against the six dreadful diseases.

(v) Activeness of the child.

(vi) His vision and hearing capacity, walking, etc.

(c) Assessment of nutritional status of a community.

In nutritional surveys the examination of a random and representative sample of the population covering all ages and both sex in different socio-economic groups is sufficient to be able to draw valid conclusions.

Assessment methods:—
1. Clinical examination.
2. Anthropometry.
3. Biochemical evaluation.
4. Functional assessment.

5. Assessment of dietary intake.
6. Vital and health statistics.
7. Ecological studies.

1. *Clinical examination:* It is an essential feature of all nutritional surveys since their ultimate objective is to assess levels of health of individuals or of population groups in relation to food they consume. There are a number of physical signs, some specific and many non-specific, known to be associated with states of malnutrition. However clinical signs have the following drawbacks:—

(a) Malnutrition cannot be quantified on the basis of clinical signs.

(b) Many deficiencies are unaccompanied by physical signs.

(c) Lack of specificity and subjective nature of most of the physical signs.

2. *Anthropometry:* Anthropometric measurements such as height, weight, skin fold thickness and arm circumference are valuable indications of nutritional status. If anthropometric measurements are recorded over a period of time, they reflect the patterns of growth and development and how individuals deviate from the average at various ages in body size, build and nutritional status.

3. *Biochemical assessment:*—

(a) Laboratory tests:—

   (i) Hb estimation: It is an important laboratory test that is carried out in nutritional surveys.

   (ii) Stool and urine: Stool should be examined for intestinal parasites. Urine should examined for albumin and sugar.

(b) *Biochemical tests:* With increasing knowledge of the metabolic functions of vitamins and minerals, assessment of nutritional status by clinical signs has given way to more precise biochemical tests.

Some biochemical tests in nutritional surveys are:—

Nutrient	Method	Normal value
Vit. A	Serum retinol	20 mcg/dl
Thiamine	Thiamine pyrophosphate (TPP) stimulation of RBC transketolase activity.	1.00-1.23 (ratio)
Riboflavin	RBC glutathione reductase activity stimulated by FAD	1.0-1.2 (ratio)
Niacin	Urine N-methyl nicotinamide	(not reliable)
	Serum folate	6.0 mcg/ml
	Red cell folate	160 mcg/ml
Vit. B_{12}	Serum Vit. B_{12} concentration	160 mg/l
Vit. C	Leucocyte ascorbic acid	15mcg/10^8cells
Vit. K	Prothrombin time	11-16 seconds

Biochemical tests are expensive and time consuming so they are usually applied in a sub-population.

4. *Functional indicators:* Functional indices of nutritional status are emerging as an important class of diagnostic tools. Some of the functional indicators are given in the table below:—

System	Nutrients
1. Structural integrity	
Erythrocyte fragility	Vit. E, Se
Capillary fragility	Vit. C
Tensile strength	Cu
2. Host defense	
Leucocyte chemotaxis	P/E, Zn
Leucocyte phagocytic capacity	P/E, Fe
Leucocyte bactericidal capacity	P/E, Fe, Se
T cell blastogenesis	P/E, Zn
Delayed cutaneous hypersensitivity	P/E, Zn
3. Hemostasis	
Prothrombin time	Vit. K
4. Reproduction	
Sperm count	Energy, Zn
5. Nerve function	
Nerve conduction	P/E, Vit. B, Vit. B_{12}
Dark adaptation	Vit. A, Zn
EEG	P/E
6. Work capacity	
Heart rate	P/E, Fe
Vasopressor response	Vit. C

5. *Assessment of dietary intake*:—

A dietary survey may be carried out by one of the following methods:—

(i) **Weighing of raw foods:** The survey team visits the house-hold and weighs all food that is going to be cooked and eaten as well as that which is wasted or discarded. The duration may vary from 1 to 21 days but commonly 7 days which is called one dietary cycle.

(ii) **Weighing of cooked food.**

(iii) **Oral questionaire method:** Inquiries are made retrospectively about the nature and quantity of foods eaten during the previous 24 to 48 hours.

The data collected has to be transformed into:—

(a) Mean intake of food in terms are cereals, pulses, vegetables, fruits, milk, meat, fish and eggs.

(b) The mean intake of nutrients per adult man value or consumption unit.

6. *Vital statistics:* An analysis of vital statistics – mortality and morbidity data – will identify groups at high risk and indicate the extent of risk to community.

7. *Assessment of ecological factors:* A study of ecological factors comprises the following:—

(i) **Food balance sheets:** In this supplies are related to census population to derive levels of food consumption in terms of per capita supply availability.

(b) **Socio-economic factors:** Are like family size, occupation, income, education, customs, cultural patterns in relation to feeding practices of children.

(c) **Health and educational services:** PHC services, feeding and immunization programmes should also be taken into consideration.

(d) Conditioning influences: These include parasitic, bacterial and viral infections which precipitate malnutrition.

Health status of under-five children can be assessed by the following methods:—

1. *Weight:* Infants born to well-fed mothers in India weigh about 3.2 kg at birth.

    Baby doubles its birth weight by 5 months of age, trebles it by 1 year. By the end of 2nd year birth weight gets quadrupled.

2. *Height:* In first year of life, the body lengths by about 50%. In the second year another 12 to 13 cms are added. After that growth is 5-6 cms every year.

3. *Head and chest circumference:* At birth, the head circumference is larger than the chest circumference.

4. *Growth chart:* It is the visible display of the child's physical growth and development, child should be weighed atleast once every month during the first year.

    Every 2 month during second year, and every 3 month thereafter till 5 to 6 years of age. When the child's weight is plotted on the growth chart at monthly intervals against his or her age, it gives *weight-for-age* growth curve.

PART B

Q.4 Describe in detail the steps to be taken in case of an outbreak of gastroenteritis in a slum area of Delhi.

Ans. Chlorination of water: Chlorination is one of the greatest advances in water purification. Various methods of chlorination are:—

(1) *Chlorine gas:* It is cheap, quick in action, efficient and easy to apply. It is applied by a special equipment called chlorinating equipment. It is the method of first choice.

(2) *Chloramines:* These are loose compounds of chlorine and ammonia. They have a less tendency to produce chlorinous taste and give a more persistent type of residual chlorine. The greatest drawbacks of chloramines is that they have a slower action than chlorine so it is not used to a great extent in water treatment.

(3) *Perchloran:* It is a calcium compound which carries 60-70% of available chlorine.

The following measures will be employed to check gastroenteritis epidemic:—

(1) *Notification:* Early notification is very important. An outbreak of gastroenteritis should be notified immediately by telegram to the district health authority, state and national health authority.

(2) *Isolation of the case:* In the hospital or in the house should be done. The contacts should be segregated and treated.

(3) *Sterilization of water:* The water supplies should be protected from contamination and immediate disinfection of those supplies which are believed to be exposed to risk of pollution. The water may be sterilized by:—

(i) Chlorination

(ii) Permanganate of potash.

(iii) Boiling.

(4) *Protection of food:* Food should be well cooked and properly protected from flies, dust, etc. Uncooked food should be avoided and no one should be allowed to handle food without thoroughly washing and disinfecting their hands.

(5) *Fly control:* By DDT, malathion spray.

(6) *Disposal of night soil:* Indiscrete defecations should be avoided or stopped. Quick and effective disposal of night soil should be done, so that flies may not come in contact with night soil.

(7) *Disinfection:* Concurrent and terminal disinfection is required. Bleaching powder can be used.

(a) Stools and vomit: All excreta and vomit should be collected in a basin and mixed with an equal quantity of 5% cresol or 3% bleaching powder. After two hours of disinfection it should be burnt or buried.

(b) Clothings and beddings: The cloth should be soaked in 2½% cresol solution for ½ an hour and then washed with soap and water.

(c) Floors and walls: The floor must be thoroughly disinfected with 5% cresol. The walls upto a height of 3 feet should be treated similarly.

(d) Cooking utensils: Disinfected by boiling for 15 minutes or keeping them in cresol solution for ½ hour before washing finally with water and soda.

(e) Hands: Dipped in 1% cresol.

8. *Vaccination.*

9. *Health education.*

Q.5 Name the diseases preventable by vaccination under the 'Universal Immunization Programme'. Discuss in detail the prevention and control of diphtheria.

Ans. National Immunization Programme:—

In May 1974, the WHO officially launched a global immunization programme, known as the Expanded Programme on Immunization (EPI) to protect all children from six vaccine preventable diseases namely:—

(a) Diphtheria.

(b) Whooping cough.

(c) Tetanus.

(d) Polio.

(e) Tuberculosis.

(f) Measles.

The programme is now called Universal Immunization Programme.

Beneficiaries	Age	Vaccine	No. of Doses	Route of Administration
Infants	6 weeks to 9 months. 9 to 12 months	DPT Polio BCG Measles	3 3 1*	Intra muscular Oral Intra dermal Subcutaneous

Children	16 to 24 months	DPT	1**	Intra muscular
		Polio	1**	Oral
	5 to 6 years	DT	1*	Intra muscular
		Typhoid	2	Subcutaneous
	10 years	Tetanus toxoid	1@	Intra muscular
			1@	Subcutaneous
	16 years	Tetanus toxoid	1@	Intra muscular
		Typhoid	1@	Subcutaneous
Pregnant women	16 to 36 weeks	Tetanus toxoid	1@	Intra muscular

*For institutional delivery.

**Booster doses

@ 2 doses, it not vaccinated.

Cold chain: The cold chain is a system of storage and transport of vaccines at low temperature from the manufacturer to the actual vaccination site. The cold chain system is necessary because vaccine failure may occur due to a failure in storing and transporting the vaccine under strict temperature controls. The cold chain equipment consist of:—

(i) Cold box: It is meant to transport large quantities of vaccine by vehicle to out of reach sites.

(ii) Vaccine carrier: It is meant to transport small quantities of vaccine by bicycle or by foot.

(iii) Flasks: They are used if vaccine carriers are not available.

(iv) Ice-packs.

(v) Refrigerator.

Prevention and control of diphtheria:—

1. Most effective preventive measure is through artificial active immunization with alum precipitated toxoid.

DPT vaccine is used against diphtheria, pertussis and tetanus. Inoculation is done at 1-3 months of age and repeated twice at 4-6 weeks intervals.

A booster dose is given at 1 year of age and then on entry into school.

Schick test: Though rarely practied, it helps to distinguish persons susceptible to diphtheria from non-susceptible ones. $1/50^{th}$ of the minimum lethal dose of diphtheria toxin is injected intradermally on the forearm with toxins heated to 75°C. Positive skin reaction indicates that there is no immunity.

2. During the outbreak of the disease:—

(i) Prompt notification.

(ii) Isolation of patient at home or hospital.

(iii) Concurrent and terminal disinfection.

(iv) Exclusion of contact children from school at least for 2 weeks.

3. The health authorities should especially concentrate on the following steps:—

(i) Careful search for clinical cases and carriers is a practically very important step.

(ii) Prompt active immunization, with precipitated toxin, of all persons not recently immunized, especially the school children and then the adults. Old people are merely kept under observation.

(iii) Search for a common source: Throats swab culture and mass Schick testing is helpful.

(iv) Prompt antitoxin in full therapeutic doses to the actual patients.

(v) Ascertain that media like milk are not serving as a vehicle fix infection.

Q.6 Discuss the epidemiology and prevention of AIDS.

Ans. Epidemiological Features:—

(a) *Agent:* (HIV) Human Immunodeficiency Virus. The virus uses the human cells to perpetuate itself. The virus replicates in actively dividing T_4 lymphocytes and to remain in lymphoid cells in a latent state that can be activated. The virus has a unique ability to destroy human T_4 help cells. The virus is able to spread throughout the body, it can pass through the blood-brain barrier and can then destroy some brain cells. The virus can be easily killed by heat, inactivated by ether, acetone, ethanol.

(b) *Reservoir of infection:* Cases and carriers. Once a person is infected, the virus remains in the body lifelong.

(c) *Source of infection:* Highest concentration of virus is found in:—

(i) Blood.

(ii) Semen.

(iii) CSF.

(d) *Age:* Most cases are between 20-49 years.

(b) *Sex:* Homosexual and bisexuals.

(c) *High Rise Groups*: Male homosexuals and bisexuals, heterosexual partners, intravenous drug abusers, transfusion recipients of blood and blood products.

(d) *Immunology:* The immune system disorders associated with HIV infection/AIDS is considered to occur primarily from the gradual depletion in a specialized group of WBC called T-helper or t-4 cells. The full name of T helper cell is the CD4 + T lymphocyte – is also commonly known as CD4 + cell. These cells play a key role in regulating the immune response.

Preventive care:—

(i) Immunization: Of the children against 6 dreadful and preventable diseases. These are diphtheria, tetanus, pertussis, measles, polio, tuberculosis.

(ii) Nutritional surveillance: It is extremely important for identifying sub-clinical nutrition. Almost all major nutritional disorders occurs in this age.

(iii) Health check-ups: Cover physical examination and should be provided every 3 to 6 months.

(iv) Oral rehydration: A poor child suffers 2 to 6 times in a year with diarrhea. The use of ORS has opened the way for a drastic reduction in child mortality and malnutrition.

(v) Family planning: In the center of symbol is a triangular area. If it is colored red we have the family planning triangle of India.

(vi) Health education: Around the whole symbol is a border that touches all areas, this border represents health teachings.

Part C

Q.7 What are the preventive measure to be undertaken at the household level in case of the following disease outbreaks:—

(a) **Hepatitis A.**

(b) **Tuberculosis.**

(c) **Cholera.**

(d) **Chicken-pox.**

(e) **Plague.**

(f) **Measles.**

Ans.(a) Hepatitis A:—

Hepatitis A is transmitted mainly by feco-oral route: It occurs by direct person to person contact or indirectly by contaminated water, food or milk.

During the outbreak of Hepatitis A, water should be treated properly before drinking and stored in a safe and clean container. The feces should be disinfected. The personal and community hygiene like hand washing before eating and after toilet; the sanitary disposal of excreta which will prevent contamination of water, food and milk; and purification of water, milk supply by flocculation, filtration and adequate chlorination.

(b) **Tuberculosis:** It is an infectious disease caused by M. tuberculosis. T.B. contiues to be a major health problem in India. Preventive measures are: A patient infected with T.B. should be isolated. All his excretions should be disinfected. We should not go very near the patient.

All the medicines should be given in time and a proper course should be done.

Patient should be given moral support, utensils and other

material used by the patient should be disinfected. The room of a T.B. patient should be disinfected with formaldehyde, spray before using. If a bovine tuberculosis outbreak has occurred, we should not take milk from gwalas but from Mother Dairy.

(c) **Cholera:** Is an acute diarrhea disease. As water is the most important vehicle for transmission of cholera, so the water should be purified before drinking by boiling, filtration and chlorination.

Excreta disposal should also be sanitary. Outdoor food habits should be restricted. Proper handling of food with sanitation. Disinfection of the stool, vomit, etc. before disposal.

(d) **Chickenpox:** Is an acute, highly infectious disease. It is characterized by vesicular rashes, fever and malaise. During a chickenpox outbreak the patient should be isolated for about 6 days after the onset of rash. Disinfection of articles soiled by nose and throat discharges should be carried out.

(e) **Plague:** During an epidemic outbreak, insecticides should be sprayed in house like DDT, BHC, etc. The most effective method is to break the chain of transmission. All patients should be isolated. Rat-traps and other antirodent measures should be used to control rats. If any rat dies in the locality or house, immediately inform to health services.

(f) **Measles:** Is a highly infections disease of childhood caused by a specific group of virus mycoviruses. The virus is transmitted by droplet infection:—

   (i) Patient should be isolated for 7 days after the onset of rashes.

   (ii) Immunization of contacts within 2 days.

(iii) Immunization of pregnant mothers during an epidemic outbreak of measles.

Q.8 Enumerate the various STDs. Discuss the role of social factors in their causation and methods to control them?

Ans. Bacterial STDs:—

(a) Gonorrhea.
(b) Genital chlamydial infection.
(c) Syphilis.
(d) Chancroid.

Viral STDs:—

Genital herpes.

Genital human papilloma.

Virus infection.

Role of social factors:—

(1) *Prostitution:* A Major factor in the spread of STDs. A prostitute acts as a reservoir of infection.
(2) *Broken families:* Due to the death of one partner or due to separation. The atmosphere in such homes is unhappy and children reared in such an atmosphere are likely to go astray in search of other avenues of happiness.
(3) *Sexual disharmony:* Married people with strained relations, divorced and separated persons are often victim of STDs.
(4) *Easy money:* It provides an occupation for easy money.
(5) *Emotional immaturity:* Social factor in acquiring STDs.

(6) *Urbanization and industrialization:* These are conductive to the type of lifestyle that contributes to high levels of infection; since long working hours, relative isolation from family and geographical and social mobility foster casual sexual relationships.

(7) *Social disruption:* Caused by disasters, war and civil unrest have always increased STDs.

(8) *International level:* Travellers can import as well as export infection.

(9) *Changed behavioral pattern:* Equal rights to both sexes, independence or idea, etc.

(10) *Social stigma:* Leads to non-detection of cases, dropping out before treatment is complete.

Control of STDs:—

1. *Case detection:—*

(i) Screening of healthy volunteers: Screening of special groups, viz. pregnant women, blood donors, industrial workers, army, police, prostitutes, etc.

(ii) Contact training: It is the term used for the technique by which sexual partners of diagnosed patients are identified, located, investigated and treated.

(iii) Cluster testing: Here the patients are asked to name others persons of either sex.

2. *Case holding and treatment:* Adequate treatment of patients and their contacts. Every effort should be made to ensure complete and adequate treatment.

3. *Epidemiological treatment:* It consists of administrating

full therapeutic dose of treatment to persons recently exposed to STD while awaiting the results of laboratory tests.

4. *Personal prophylaxis:—*

(i) Contraceptives.

(ii) Vaccines for hepatitis B.

5. *Health education:* Principal aim of educational intervention is to help individuals alter their behaviour in an effort to avoid STDs, that is to minimize disease acquisition and transmission.

Q.9 What is primary health care? How is this care delivered in our country? Discuss in detail.

Ans. Primary health care is based on the principal of "placing people's health in people's hand" to achieve the goal of *health for all* which the Government of India has started primary health care which seeks to provide universal, comprehensive health care at a cost which people can afford.

1. **Village level:** We have:—

(a) Village health guides.

(b) Training of local dais.

(c) ICDS scheme.

(a) *Village health guides:* The health guides are now mostly women. The health guides come from and are chosen by the community in which they work. They serve as links between the community and the government. Health guides recieve a working manual and a kit of simple medicines belonging to the modern and traditional systems. Duty of health guides include treatment of simple medicinal ailments and activities in first aid, mother and child health including family planning, health education and sanitation.

(b) *Local dais:* The training for local dais is for 30 working days. Each dai is paid a stipend of Rs. 300 during the training period. Training is given at the PHC, subcentre or MCH center for 2 days and the remaining 4 days they accompany a health worker. During her training, each dai is required to conduct at least 2 deliveries in the guidance of a health worker (F).

(c) *Aganwadi worker:* There is one aganwadi worker for 1000 population. She undergoes training and after that she is given Rs. 200-250 per month for services she renderes like nutrition, health and education, checkup, immunization, supplementary nutrition.

Beneficiaries are women (15-45 years) and children (1-4 years).

2. Sub-centre level: One sub-center for each 5000 population in general and one sub-centre for each 3000 population in hilly areas. Each sub-center is limited to the function of mother and child care, family planning and immunization.

Staff at a sub-centre level:—

Health worker (female)/ANM	1
Health worker (male)	1
Voluntary worker	1
	3

3. Primary health center:—

The Bhore committee in 1946 gave the concept of primary health center as a basic health unit, to provide, as close to the people as possible, an integrated curative and preventive health care to rural population with emphasis on preventive and promotive aspects of health care.

One PHC for every 30,000 rural populations in the plains and one PHC for every 20,000 population in hilly, tribal and backward area.

Function of PHC:—

(i) Medical care.

(ii) MCH including family planning.

(iii) Safe water and basic sanitation.

(iv) Prevention and control of locally endemic diseases.

(v) Collection and reporting of vital statistics.

(vi) Education about health.

(vii) National health Programmes.

(viii) Referral services.

(ix) Training of health guides, health workers, local dais and health assistants.

(x) Basic laboratory services.

Staffing pattern at PHC level:—

Medical officer	1
Pharmacist	1
Nurses/midwife	1
Health worker (female)	1
Block extension educator	1
Health assistant (male)	1
Health assistant (female)	1
UDC	1
LDC	1
Lab technician	1
Driver	1
Class IV	4
Total	15

II B.H.M.S. 2000

PART A

Q.1 Plan health education activities for control of an epidemic of gastroenteritis in Delhi?

Ans. Chlorination of water: Chlorination is one of the greatest advances in water purification. Various methods of chlorination are:—

(1) *Chlorine gas:* It is cheap, quick in action, efficient and easy to apply. It is applied by a special equipment called chlorinating equipment. It is the method of first choice.

(2) *Chloramines:* These are loose compounds of chlorine and ammonia. They have a less tendency to produce chlorinous taste and give a more persistent type of residual chlorine. The greatest drawbacks of chloramines is that they have a slower action than chlorine so it is not used to a great extent in water treatment.

(3) *Perchloran:* It is a calcium compound which carries 60-70% of available chlorine.

The following measures will be employed to check gastroenteritis epidemic:—

(1) *Notification:* Early notification is very important. An outbreak of gastroenteritis should be notified immediately by telegram to the district health authority, state and national health authority.

(2) *Isolation of the case:* In the hospital or in the house should be done. The contacts should be segregated and treated.

(3) *Sterilization of water:* The water supplies should be protected from contamination and immediate disinfection of those supplies which are believed to be exposed to risk of pollution. The water may be sterilized by:—

(i) Chlorination

(ii) Permanganate of potash.

(iii) Boiling.

(4) *Protection of food:* Food should be well cooked and properly protected from flies, dust, etc. Uncooked food should be avoided and no one should be allowed to handle food without thoroughly washing and disinfecting their hands.

(5) *Fly control:* By DDT, malathion spray.

(6) *Disposal of night soil:* Indiscrete defecations should be avoided or stopped. Quick and effective disposal of night soil should be done, so that flies may not come in contact with night soil.

(7) *Disinfection:* Concurrent and terminal disinfection is required. Bleaching powder can be used.

(a) Stools and vomit: All excreta and vomit should be collected in a basin and mixed with an equal quantity of 5% cresol or 3%

bleaching powder. After two hours of disinfection it should be burnt or buried.

(b) Clothings and beddings: The cloth should be soaked in 2½% cresol solution for ½ an hour and then washed with soap and water.

(c) Floors and walls: The floor must be thoroughly disinfected with 5% cresol. The walls upto a height of 3 feet should be treated similarly.

(d) Cooking utensils: Disinfected by boiling for 15 minutes or keeping them in cresol solution for ½ hour before washing finally with water and soda.

(e) Hands: Dipped in 1% cresol.

   8. *Vaccination.*

   9. *Health education.*

Q.2 Enumerate nutritional programmes and describe the mid-day meal programme in detail.

Ans. Nutritional programmes are:—

1. Vitamin A prophylaxis programme.

2. Prophylaxis against nutritional anemia.

3. Control of iodine deficiency disorders.

4. Specific nutrition programme.

5. Balwadi nutrition programme.

6. ICDS programme.

7. Mid-day meal programme.

Mid-day meal programme:—

Mid-day meal programme: Is in operation since 1961 throughout the country. The major objective of the programme is to attract more children for admission to schools and retain them so that literacy among children could be improved. The following broad principle should be kept in mind:

(a) The meals should be a supplement and not a substitute to the home diet.
(b) The meal should supply at least one-third of the total the energy requirement and half the protein needed.
(c) The cost of the meal should be reasonably low.
(d) The meal should be such that it can be prepared easily in schools.
(e) As far as possible locally available food should be used.
(f) The men should be changed frequently to avoid monotony.

Q.3 Write the primary prevention of:—

(a) **CHD.**
(b) **Hypertension.**
(c) **Cancer.**
(d) **Diabetes Mellitus.**
(e) **Obesity.**

Ans. (a) CHD: Personality which is prone to CHD is mesomorphic, aggressive, hard driving, restless with staccato speech. He is competitive.

Predisposing risk factors for CHD are:—

1. Hypertension.
2. Heavy smoking.
3. Diabetes mellitus.
4. Mental stress.
5. Obesity.
6. Excessive intake of saturated fats, cholesterol and alcohol.
7. Thyrotoxicosis.
8. Sedentary habits, lack of regular exercise and irregular ways of life.
9. Gout.

Preventive and control measures:—

1. Population strategy or primary prevention.
   (i) Prevention in whole population.
   (ii) Primordial prevention.
2. High risk strategy.
3. Secondary prevention.

1. Population strategy or primary prevention:—
(i) Prevention in whole population: Include following specific interventions:—
(a) Dietary changes:—
- Reduction of fat intake to 20-30%.
- Consumption of saturated fatty acid must be limited to less than 10% of total energy intake.

- A reduction of dietary cholesterol to below 100 mg per 1000 Kcal per day.
- An increase in complex carbohydrate consumption.
- Avoidance of alcohol consumption; reduction of salt intake to 5g daily or less.

(b) Smoking: The goal is to achieve a smokeless society.

(c) B.P.: Even a small reduction in the average B.P. of the whole population by a mere 2 to 3 mm Hg would produce a large reduction in the incidence of cardiovascular complications.

(d) Physical activity: Regular physical activity should be a part of normal daily life.

(ii) Premordial prevention: It involves preventing the emergence and spread of CHD risk factors and lifestyles that have not yet appeared or become endemic.

2. High risk strategy:—

(i) Identifying the risk: By simple tests such as B.P. and serum cholesterol measurements.

(ii) Specific advice: The next step is to bring them under preventive care and motivate them into taking a positive action against all the identified risk factors.

3. Secondary prevention: Are like drug trials, coronary surgery, use of pace makers and all the preventive measures discussed above.

(b) Hypertension: May be primary (essential) whose exact etiology is not known or secondary in which factors for hypertension are renal, adrenal gland tumors, toxemias of pregnancy, etc.

Predisposing factors:—

1. Hereditary and familial tendency.
2. Obesity.
3. Stress and strains in life.
4. Worry and nervous tension.
5. Overeating esp. saturated fats and high salt intake.
6. Alcohol smoking, tobacco chewing.

Prevention and control measures:—

1. There must be a routine B.P. record of every patient.
2. Heavy smoking and excessive alcohol drinking should be avoided.
3. One should learn to live with unavoidable worry, tension and strain in life.
4. Proper diet control.
5. All these factors should be stressed on the public through health education, primary health centers.

(c) Cancer: The etiology of cancer is not known exactly.

Contributory agent factors:—

1. Chemical agents
   - Organic – Coal tar, aniline dyes, etc.
   - Inorganic – Asbestos, nickel, etc.
2. Physical agents eg., X-ray, ultra violet rays and radiations.
3. Nutritional agents eg., polyunsaturated fats when kept for

long as such or after heating are oxidized and tend to develop mutagenic and carcinogenic substances.

    4. Mechanical agents eg., friction, trauma, etc.

Contributory factors in man:—

1. Age: Incidence of cancer is more with advance in age although some cancers like leukemia occur in young as well.
2. Sex: Lung and esophageal cancer → males.
         Breast cancer → females.
3. Some cancers are associated with the occupation.
4. Hereditary and environmental factors.

Prevention and control:—

1. Try to avoid and protect against known carcinogenic agents.
2. Ensure proper personal hygiene.
3. Health education.
4. Early cancer detection. People should also have awareness about salient features which need detection and investigation. These are: chronic swelling, lump in breast, hoarseness, excessive menstrual bleeding.
5. Persons in old age should be encouraged and motivated for regular medical checkups

(d) Diabetes mellitus: Clinical diabetes is manifested by hyperglycemia and glycosuria due to deficient or lack of insulin secretion or its ineffectiveness which results in impaired metabolism of the nutrients.

Prevention and control:—

1. Detection of prediabetic cases, which show impaired glucose tolerance curve.
2. Diet control.
3. Maintenance of standard weight.
4. Known diabetics should be motivated for proper treatment and maintenance.
5. Proper health education.

(e) Obesity: Common causes are:—

Overeating and sedentary habits.

Prevention:—

1. No overeating.
2. Regular daily exercise.
3. Avoid saturated fats, sugar.
4. No eating between the meals.
5. No alcohol.
6. Dietary therapy preferred to so called drug therapy.

PART B

Q.4 Enumerate food borne diseases and discuss epidemic dropsy in detail.

Ans. Food borne diseases:—

A. *Food borne intoxications:—*

1. Due to naturally occurring toxins in some foods:

    (a) Lathyrism.

    (b) Endemic ascites.

2. Due to toxins produced by certain bacteria:—

    (a) Botulism.

    (b) Staphylococcus poisons.

3. Due to toxins produced by some fungi:—

    (a) Aflatoxin.

    (b) Ergot.

    (c) Fusalium toxins.

4. Food borne chemical poisoning:—

    (a) Heavy metals eg., mercury, cadmium and lead.

    (b) Dils, petroleum derivatives.

    (c) Migrant chemicals from packages.

    (d) Asbestos.

    (e) Pesticide residues.

B. *Food borne infections:—*

1. Bacterial diseases:—

    (a) Typhoid fever.

    (b) Paratyphoid fever.

    (c) Salmonellosis.

    (d) Staphylococcal intoxication.

    (e) Botulism.

2. Viral diseases:—

    (a) Viral hepatitis.

    (b) Gastroenteritis.

3. Parasites:—

    (a) Taeniasis.

    (b) Trichinosis.

    (c) Ascariasis.

    (d) Amoebiasis.

Epidemic dropsy: It is caused due to contamination of mustard oil with argemone oil. There is a toxic alkaloid *Sanguinarine* from argemone oil. This toxic substance interferes with the oxidation of pyruvic acid which accumulates in the blood.

The symptoms are:—

Sudden non-inflammatory, bilateral swelling of legs, often associated with diarrhea. Dyspnea, cardiac failure and death may follow.

Contamination occur accidentally or deliberately. Seeds of argemone resemble mustard seeds. Crops of mustard are gathered in March and during this season argemone also matures and is likely to be harvested along with mustard seeds. Sometimes dealers mix argemone oil with mustard oil.

Tests may be applied for detection of argemone oil:—

(1) *Nitric acid test:* A simple test is to add nitric acid to the sample of oil in the test tube. The tube is shaken and the appearance of a brown to orange-red colour shows argemone oil.

(2) *Paper chromatography test.*

Q.5 What are the diseases transmitted by houseflies? Discuss their prevention and control measures.

Ans. Diseases transmitted by houseflies are:—

(a) Typhoid and paratyphoid fevers.

(b) Diarrheas.

(c) Dysenteries.

(d) Cholera.

(e) Gastroentritis.

(f) Amoebiasis.

(g) Helminthic infestations.

(h) Poliomyelitis.

(i) Conjunctivitis.

(j) Trachoma.

(k) Anthrax.

(l) Yaws.

Fly control measures:—

(a) *Environmental control:—*

(i) Storing garbage, kitchen wastes and other refuse in bins with tight lids.

(ii) Efficient collection, removal and disposal of refuse by incineration, compositing and sanitary land fill.

(iii) Provision of sanitary latrines.

(iv) Stopping open air defecation.

(v) Sanitary disposal of animal excreta.

(b) *Insecticidal control:—*

(i) Residual sprays: DDT, lindane, fenthion, malathion. The addition of sugar to insecticidal formulations enhances their effectiveness.

(ii) Baits: Poisoned baits contain 1 or 2 percent diazinon, malathion; liquid baits contain 0.1 to 0.2% of same insecticides and 10% sugar water. The cheapest bait is one that is made by mixing 3 teaspoons of formalin with one pint of H_2O.

(iii) Cords and ribbons: Impregnated with diazinon, fenthion have been tried with success.

(iv) Space sprays contain pyrethrin, DDT or HCH.

(c) *Fly papers:—*

It is made by the mixing of zib resin and one put of castor oil. It is heated until the mixture resembles molasses. This is smeared on paper by using an ordinary paint brush.

(d) *Protection against flies:* Screaning of houses, hosptitals, food markets, etc. Screens with meshes to the inch will keep out houseflies.

(e) *Health education.*

Q.6 Write short notes on:—

(a) **Sanitary latrine.**

(b) **Household methods for purification of water.**

(c) **Disinfection of wells.**

Ans. (a) **Sanitary latrine:—**

Non-service type:—

(a) Bore hole latrine.
(b) Dug well or pit latrine.
(c) Water seal type of latrines.

    (i) P.R.A.I. type.
    (ii) R.C.A. type.
    (iii) Sulabh shauchalya.

(d) Septic tank.
(e) Aqua privy.

We will recommend the water seal type latrine in rural areas.

Essential features of R.C.A. latrine are described below:—

(1) *Location:* It should not be located within 15 m from a source

of water supply, it should be at a lower elevation to prevent bacterial contamination of water supply.

(2) *Squatting plate:* It should be made of impervious material so that it can be washed and kept completely dry.

(3) *Pan:* Retrieves night soil urine and wash water. The length of pan is 17 inches. The width of the front portion of the pan is minimum 5 inches and width at its widest part is 8 inches.

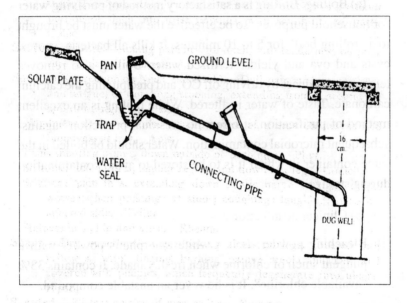

(4) *Trap:* It is a bent pipe about 7.5 cm in diameter and is connected with the pan. It holds the water and provides necessary "water seal". It is a distance between the level of water in the trap and the lowest point in the concave upper surface of the trap. Water seal is 2 cm and it prevents the access by flies and suppresses the nuisance from smell.

(5) *Connecting pipes:* When the pit is dug away from the squatting plate so connecting pipes are required to join them.

(6) *Dug well:* Or pit is usually deep and is covered.

(7) *Superstructure:* It is used to provide privacy.

(b) Household methods for purification of water.

Three methods are generally available for purifying water on a small scale. These methods can be used singly or in combination.

(a) Boiling: Boiling is a satisfactory method of purifying water for household purposes. To be effective the water must be brought to a "rolling boil" for 5 to 10 minutes. It kills all bacteria, spores, cysts and ova and yields sterilized water. Boiling also removes temporary hardness by driving off CO_2 and precipitating the calcium carbonate. Taste of water is altered. While boiling is an excellent method of purification, it offers no "residual protection" against subsequent microbial contamination. Water should be boiled in the same container in which it is to be stored to avoid contamination during storage.

(b) Clinical disinfections:—

(i) Bleaching powder: It is a white amorphous powder with a pungent smell of chlorine when freshly made. It contains 33% "available chlorine". It is however an unstable compound.

On exposure to light, air it looses its chlorine content. But when mixed with excess of lime, it retains its strength, this is called "stabilized lime."

(ii) Chlorine solution: May be prepared from bleaching powder. If 4 kgs of bleaching powder with 25% available chlorine is mixed with 20 litres of water it will give 5% solution of chlorine.

(iii) High test hypochlorite: These are calcium compounds which contains 60-70% available chlorine. It is more stable than bleaching powder and deteriorates much less on storage.

(iv) Chlorine tablets: These are available in the market under various trade-names (viz. halozone tablets). They are quite good for disinfecting small quantities of water.

(v) Iodine: Two drops of 2% ethanol solution of iodine will suffice for one litre of clear water. A contact time of 20 to 30 minutes is needed for effective disinfections.

(vi) Potassium permanganate: Although a powerful oxidizing agent, it is not a satisfactory agent for disinfecting water. It may kill cholera vibrios, but is of little use against other disease organisms. It alters the color, smell and taste of water.

(c) Filteration:—

Water can be purified on a small scale by filtering through ceramic filters such as Pasteur Chamberland filter, Berkefeld filter

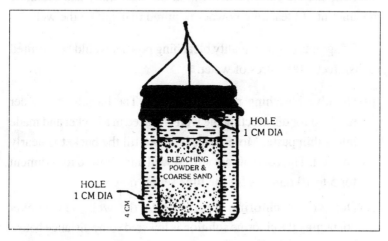

and Katadyn filter. The essential part of filter is the "candle" which is made of porcelain in the Chamberland type and of kieselgurh in the Berkefeld filter.

(c) Disinfection of wells:—

The most effective and cheapest method of disinfecting wells is by bleaching powder.

Steps in well disinfection:—

(i) Find the volume of water in the well.

    (a) Measure the depth of water column —— (h) meter
    (b) Measure the diameter of well —— (d) metres
    (c) Substitute h and d in

$$V = \frac{3.14 \times d^2 \times h}{4} \times 100$$

    (d) One cubic metre = 1000 litres of water.

(ii) Find the amount of bleaching powder required for disinfection.

Estimate the chlorine demand of the well water and calculate the amount of bleaching powder required to disinfect the well.

2.5 grams of good quality bleaching powder would be required to disinfect 1,000 litres of water.

(iii) Dissolve bleaching powder in water: The bleaching powder required for disinfecting the well is placed in a bucket and made into a thin paste. More water is added till the bucket is nearly ¾th full. The contents are stirred well and allowed to sediment for 5 to 10 minutes for the lime settles down.

(iv) Delivery of chlorine solution into the well. The bucket containing the chlorine solution is lowered some distance below the water surface and the well water is agitated by moving the bucket violently both vertically and laterally.

(v) Contact period should be 1 hour.

(vi) Ortho-tolicline Arsenite Test.

It is a good practice to test for residual chlorine at the end of one hour contact. If the free chlorine level is less than 0.5 mg/litre, the chlorination procedure should be repeated.

Q.7 Discuss the National Tuberculosis Control Programme.

Ans. The National Tuberculosis Programme: It has been in operation since 1962. The goal of NTP is to reduce the problem of tuberculosis in the community sufficiently quickly to the level where it ceases to be a public health problem.

District Tuberculosis Programme (DTP) is the backbone of NTP. The District Tuberculosis Centre (DTC) is the nucleus to DTP. The function of the DTC is to plan, organize and implement the DTP in the entire district in association with general health services.

Their activities include:—

(a) *Case finding:* Sputum examination is done to detect new T.B. cases in rural population. To further improve case finding male health workers are required to collect and fix sputum of the symptomatic cases on the slide during their routine visits to the villages and send the slides to the nearest health center for microscopic examination.

(b) *Treatment:* It is free and is offered on domiciliary basis from all the health institutions. It is organized in such a manner that patients are expected to collect drugs once a month on fixed dates from the nearest treatment centre. When the patient fails to collect his/her drugs on the "due date", a letter is written to him/her and in the event of no response for 7 days a home visit is paid by the hospital staff.

(c) *BCG vaccination:* By UIP, the coverage of BCG has gone up.

(d) *Recording and reporting:* The names and addresses of all the sputum the cases are sent to DTC every Saturday. The DTC registers all sputum positive cases.

(e) *Supervision:* The DTC team visits the peripheral health institutions regularly and helps them in planning and rendering T.B. control services.

The DTC team includes:—

1 District tuberculosis officer.

1 Laboratory technician.

1 Treatment organiser.

1 X-ray technician.

1 Non-medical team leader.

1 Statistical assistant.

Prevention and control of T. B.:—

1. It should be a compulsorily notifiable disease.
2. All the sputum positive patients should be isolated till they are sputum negative.
3. All detected cases should be promptly treated with a proper follow up to ensure the continuity of their treatment.

4. Chemoprophylaxis of all known contacts should be undertaken.
5. Early diagnosis and detection of cases.
6. Rehabilitation of the treated cases.
7. Health education of the public so that they should endeavour to avoid exposure to infection and cooperate in BCG vaccination and chemoprophylaxis, etc.
8. Some of the practical methods under the mass screening programme are as follows:—

(i) Mass tuberculin testing is useful in establishing index of infection in a given community.

(ii) Sputum examination for AFB. This is one of the easiest and fruitful methods to uncover many undetected tubercular cases.

(iii) BCG vaccination should be given to new borns below four weeks and the other susceptible individuals to protect against the infection.

Q.8 Write short notes on:—

(a) IMR.

(b) MMR.

(c) National Immunization Programme.

Ans.(a) IMR: It is defined as the ratio of infant death registered in a given year to the total number of live births registered in the same year, usually expressed as a rate per 1000 live births.

$$IMR = \frac{\text{Number of deaths of children less than 1 year of age in a year}}{\text{Number of live births in same year}} \times 1000$$

(b) MMR: It is defined as death of a woman when pregnant or within 42 days of termination of pregnancy, irrespective of the duration and site of pregnancy from any cause related or aggravated by pregnancy.

$$\frac{\text{Total number of female deaths due to complications of pregnancy, child birth or within 42 days if delivery from puerperal causes in an area during a given year}}{\text{Total no. of live birth in same year.}} \times 1000$$

Causes:—

1. Toxemias of pregnancy.
2. Hemorrhage.
3. Infection.
4. Induced abortion.
5. Obstructed labor.
6. Anemia.
7. Other related diseases eg., cardiac, renal, etc.

Prevention:—

1. Dietary supplementation.
2. Prevention of infection and hemorrhage.
3. Prevention of complications eg., eclampsia, malpresentations.
4. Treatment of medical conditions eg., hypertension.
5. Promotion of family planning.
6. Anti-malaria and tetanus prophylaxis.

(c) National Immunization Programme:—

In May 1974, the WHO officially launched a global immunization programme, known as the Expanded Programme on Immunization (EPI) to protect all children from six vaccine preventable diseases namely:—

(a) Diphtheria.
(b) Whooping cough.
(c) Tetanus.
(d) Polio.
(e) Tuberculosis.
(f) Measles.

The programme is now called Universal Immunization Programme.

Beneficiaries	Age	Vaccine	No. of Doses	Route of Administration
Infants	6 weeks to 9 months. 9 to 12 months	DPT Polio BCG Measles	3 3 1*	Intra muscular Oral Intra dermal Subcutaneous
Children	16 to 24 months 5 to 6 years 10 years 16 years	DPT Polio DT Typhoid Tetanus toxoid Tetanus toxoid Typhoid	1** 1** 1* 2 1@ 1@ 1@ 1@	Intra muscular Oral Intra muscular Subcutaneous Intra muscular Subcutaneous Intra muscular Subcutaneous
Pregnant women	16 to 36 weeks	Tetanus toxoid	1@	Intra muscular

*For institutional delivery.

**Booster doses

@ 2 doses, it not vaccinated.

Cold chain: The cold chain is a system of storage and transport of vaccines at low temperature from the manufacturer to the actual vaccination site. The cold chain system is necessary because vaccine failure may occur due to a failure in storing and transporting the vaccine under strict temperature controls. The cold chain equipment consist of:—

(i) Cold box: It is meant to transport large quantities of vaccine by vehicle to out of reach sites.

(ii) Vaccine carrier: It is meant to transport small quantities of vaccine by bicycle or by foot.

(iii) Flasks: They are used if vaccine carriers are not available.

(iv) Ice-packs.

(v) Refrigerator.

Q.9 Write short notes on:—

(a) Functions of PHC

(b) Under-five clinic.

(c) Anti-larval measures for control of mosquities.

Ans.(a) Functions of PHC:—

The Bhore committee in 1946 gave the concept of primary health center as a basic health unit, to provide, as close to the people as possible, an integrated curative and preventive health care to rural population with emphasis on preventive and promotive aspects of health care.

One PHC for every 30,000 rural populations in the plains and one PHC for every 20,000 population in hilly, tribal and backward area.

Function of PHC:—

(i) Medical care.
(ii) MCH including family planning.
(iii) Safe water and basic sanitation.
(iv) Prevention and control of locally endemic diseases.
(v) Collection and reporting of vital statistics.
(vi) Education about health.
(vii) National health Programmes.
(viii) Referral services.
(ix) Training of health guides, health workers, local dais and health assistants.
(x) Basic laboratory services.

Staffing pattern at PHC level:—

Medical officer	1
Pharmacist	1
Nurses/midwife	1
Health worker (female)	1
Block extension educator	1
Health assistant (male)	1

Health assistant (female)	1
UDC	1
LDC	1
Lab technician	1
Driver	1
Class IV	4
Total	**15**

(b) Under-fives clinic:—

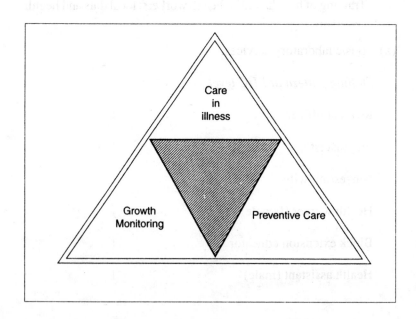

Under-five clinic offers a blend of curative, preventive and promotive health services within the resources available in the country, making use of non-professional auxillaries, thus making the services not only economical but also available to a larger proportion of children in the community.

Aims and objectives:—

The aims and objectives of under-five clinic are set out in the symbol or emblem:—

1. Care in illness:—

The apex of the symbol represents "care and treatment of sick children"; care of sick children can be handled by trained nurses.

The illness care for children will comprise of:—

(a) Diagnosis and treatment of:—
   (i) Acute illness.
   (ii) Chronic illness including physical, mental, congenital and acquired abnormalities.
   (iii) Disorders of growth and development.
(b) X-ray and laboratory services.
(c) Referral services.

2. Preventive care:—

(i) Immunization: Of the children against 6 dreadful and preventable diseases. These are diphtheria, tetanus, pertussis, measles, polio, tuberculosis.

(ii) Nutritional surveillance: It is extremely important for identifying sub-clinical nutrition. Almost all major nutritional disorders occurs in this age.

(iii) Health check-ups: Cover physical examination and should be provided every 3 to 6 months.

(iv) Oral rehydration: A poor child suffers 2 to 6 times in a year with diarrhea. The use of ORS has opened the way for a drastic reduction in child mortality and malnutrition.

(v) Family planning: In the center of symbol is a triangular area. If it is colored red we have the family planning triangle of India.

(vi) Health education: Around the whole symbol is a border that touches all areas, this border represents health teachings.

3. Growth monitoring:—

It is to weigh the child periodically at monthly intervals during the first year, every 2 months, during the second year, and every 3 months thereafter up to the age of 5 to 6 years when the child's weight is plotted against his or her age as it gives the *growth curve.*

(c) Antilarval measures for control of mosquitoes:—

(a) Environmental control: Reducing their breeding places. This is known as source reduction and comprises of minor engineering methods such as filling, leveling and drainage of breeding places:—

Culex: Reducing domestic and predomestic sources of breeding such as cesspools and open ditches.

Aedes: Environment should be cleaned up and got rid of water holding containers such as discarded tins, empty pots, broken bottles, etc.

Anopheles: Breeding places should be looked for and abolished by appropriate engineering measures.

Mansonia: Reduce the aquatic plants.

(b) Chemical control: Commonly used larvicides are:—

   (i) Mineral oils.

   (ii) Paris green.

   (iii) Synthetic insecticides.

Mineral oils: The application of oil to water is one of the oldest known mosquito control measures. Since the life cycle of a mosquito occupies about 8 days or so it is customary to apply oil once a week on all breeding places.

Paris green: It is a stomach poison and to be effective it must be ingested by the larvae. Anopheles are surface feeders so it is easily killed by Paris green and for bottom feeders Paris green is applied in granular formation.

Synthetic insecticides: E.g., fenthion, chlorpyrifos and abate are effective larvicides. These organophosphorus compounds hydrolyze quickly in water.

(c) Biological control: A wide range of small fish feed readily on mosquito larvae. The best known are Gambusia offense and Lebister reticulatus.

II B.H.M.S. 2001

PART A

Q.1 Discuss the levels of prevention giving suitable examples.

Ans. Levels of prevention:—

1. Primary prevention
2. Secondary prevention.
3. Tertiary prevention.

Primary prevention: It can be defined as action taken prior to the onset of disease, which removes the possibility that disease will ever occur. It signifies the intervention in the prepathogenesis phase or a disease or health problem.

Primary prevention may be accomplished by measures designed to promote general health, well-being & quality of life in people or by specific protective measures.

The WHO has recommended the following approaches for primary prevention of chronic diseases:—

(a) Premordial prevention: Prevention of the emergence or development of risk factors in countries or population groups in which they have not yet appealed. For e.g., smoking, eating patterns.

(b) **Population (mass) Strategy:** It is directed at the whole population irrespective of individual risk factors. For e.g., studies have shown that even a small reduction in the average blood pressure of a population would produce a large reduction in cardiovascular diseases.

(c) **High-risk strategy:** It aims to bring preventive care to individuals at special risk. This requires detection of individuals at high risk by optimum use of clinical methods.

Secondary prevention: "Action which halts the progress of a disease at its incipient stage & prevents complications".

The specific interventions are:—

(a) Early diagnosis (e.g., screening tests, case finding programmes).
(b) Adequate treatment.

By early diagnosis and adequate treatment, secondary prevention attempts to arrest the disease process, restore health by seeking out unrecognized disease and treating it before reversible pathological changes have taken place.

3. *Tertiary prevention:* It signifies intervention in the late pathogenesis phase. Tertiary prevention can be defined as all measures available to reduce or limit impairments and disabilities. For e.g., treatment even if undertaken late in the natural history of a disease may prevent the sequelae and limit disability.

Modes of intervention:—
(i) Health Promotion.
(ii) Specific Protection.
(iii) Early diagnosis and treatment.

(iv) Disability limitation.

(v) Rehabilitation.

(i) *Health promotion:* It is the process of enabling people to increase control over and to improve health. It is not directed against any particular disease, but is intended to strengthen the host through a variety of approaches (interventions). The well known interventions in this area are:—

(a) Health education.
(b) Environmental modifications.
(c) Nutritional interventions.
(d) Lifestyle and behavioral changes.

(a) Health education: A large number of diseases could be prevented if people are adequately informed about them and if they are encouraged to take necessary precautions in time.

(b) Environmental modifications: Such as provision of safe water; installation of sanitary latrines; control of insects and rodents; improvement of housing, etc.

(c) Nutritional interventions: These comprise of food distribution and nutritional improvement of vulnerable groups, child feeding programmes, food fortifications, nutritional education, etc.

(d) Lifestyle and behavioral changes: The action of prevention in this case is one of individual and community responsibility for health. The physician and each health worker acts as an educator, rather than a therapist.

(ii) *Specific protection:* To avoid disease altogether is the ideal 2but this is possible only in a limited number of cases. The following are some of the currently available interventions aimed at specific protection:—

(a) Immunization.

(b) Use of specific nutrients.

(c) Chemoprophylaxis.

(d) Protection against occupational diseases.

(e) Protection against accidents.

(f) Protection against carcinogens.

(g) Avoidance of allergens.

(h) The control of specific hazards in general environment.

(iii) *Early diagnosis and treatment:* Are main interventions of disease control. The earlier a disease is diagnosed and treated the better it is from the point of view of prognosis and preventing the occurrence of further cases or any longterm disability.

(iv) *Disability limitation:* When a patient reports late in the pathogenesis phase the mode of intervention is disability limitation.

Concept of disability:—

Disease

↓

Impairment

↓

Disability

↓

Handicap

Impairment: Any loss or abnormality of psychological, physiological or anatomical structure or functions.

E.g., loss of foot, defective vision.

Disability: Because of an impairment, the affected person may be unable to carry out certain activities considered normal for his age, sex, etc.

Handicap: It is defined as a disadvantage for a given individual, resulting from an impairment or a disability that limits or prevents the fulfillment of a role that is normal.

(v) *Rehabilitation:* Defined as the combined and coordinated use of medical, social, educational and vocational measures for training and retraining the individual to the highest possible level of functional ability.

A chronic disease of national importance in India is Tuberculosis.

Primary prevention:—

(a) Premordial prevention: Discouraging the emergence or development of risk factors in the country like air pollution, crowding of houses, smoking, eating roadside food, etc.

(b) Populations strategy: Changing the lifestyle like development of socio-economic status, health education about T.B., regular check-ups, vaccination (BCG) to the children under EPI.

(c) High risk strategy: Preventive care to individuals at risk like doctors, detection of high risk groups by clinical methods, contacts of T.B. cases, nurses, etc.

Secondary prevention:—

Early diagnosis and treatment by screening tests and case finding programmes.

Case finding is done by:—

(i) Sputum examination by primary health centre workers.
(ii) Tuberculin test.

Treatment is by chemotherapy. The objective of treatment is elimination of both fast and slowly multiplying bacilli.

Teritary prevention: It is done to limit the damage to the lungs or other organs due to T.B.

Q.2 How will you assess the nutritional status of a community? Describe the measures to be taken at a community level to prevent malnutrition.

Ans. Nutritional survey: In nutritional surveys the examination of a random and representative sample of the population covering all ages and both sex in different socio-economic groups is sufficient to be able to draw valid conclusions.

Assessment methods:—

1. Clinical examination.
2. Anthropometry.
3. Biochemical evaluation.
4. Functional assessment.
5. Assessment of dietary intake.
6. Vital and health statistics.

7. Ecological studies.

1. *Clinical examination:* It is an essential feature of all nutritional surveys since their ultimate objective is to assess levels of health of individuals or of population groups in relation to food they consume. There are a number of physical signs, some specific and many non-specific, known to be associated with states of malnutrition. However clinical signs have the following drawbacks:—

(a) Malnutrition cannot be quantified on the basis of clinical signs.

(b) Many deficiencies are unaccompanied by physical signs.

(c) Lack of specificity and subjective nature of most of the physical signs.

2. *Anthropometry:* Anthropometric measurements such as height, weight, skin fold thickness and arm circumference are valuable indications of nutritional status. If anthropometric measurements are recorded over a period of time, they reflect the patterns of growth and development and how individuals deviate from the average at various ages in body size, build and nutritional status.

3. *Biochemical assessment:*—

(a) Laboratory tests:—

   (i) Hb estimation: It is an important laboratory test that is carried out in nutritional surveys.

   (ii) Stool and urine: Stool should be examined for intestinal parasites. Urine should examined for albumin and sugar.

(b) **Biochemical tests:** With increasing knowledge of the metabolic functions of vitamins and minerals, assessment of nutritional status by clinical signs has given way to more precise biochemical tests.

Some biochemical tests in nutritional surveys are:—

Nutrient	Method	Normal value
Vit. A	Serum retinol	20 mcg/dl
Thiamine	Thiamine pyrophosphate (TPP) stimulation of RBC transketolase activity.	1.00-1.23 (ratio)
Riboflavin	RBC glutathione reductase activity stimulated by FAD	1.0-1.2 (ratio)
Niacin	Urine N-methyl nicotinamide	(not reliable)
	Serum folate	6.0 mcg/ml
	Red cell folate	160 mcg/ml
Vit. B_{12}	Serum Vit. B_{12} concentration	160 mg/l
Vit. C	Leucocyte ascorbic acid	15 mcg/10^8 cells
Vit. K	Prothrombin time	11-16 seconds

Biochemical tests are expensive and time consuming so they are usually applied in a sub-population.

4. *Functional indicators:* Functional indices of nutritional status are emerging as an important class of diagnostic tools. Some of the functional indicators are given in the table below:—

System	Nutrients
1. Structural integrity	
Erythrocyte fragility	Vit. E, Se
Capillary fragility	Vit. C
Tensile strength	Cu
2. Host defense	
Leucocyte chemotaxis	P/E, Zn
Leucocyte phagocytic capacity	P/E, Fe
Leucocyte bactericidal capacity	P/E, Fe, Se
T cell blastogenesis	P/E, Zn
Delayed cutaneous hypersensitivity	P/E, Zn
3. Hemostasis	
Prothrombin time	Vit. K
4. Reproduction	
Sperm count	Energy, Zn
5. Nerve function	
Nerve conduction	P/E, Vit. B, Vit. B_{12}
Dark adaptation	Vit. A, Zn
EEG	P/E
6. Work capacity	
Heart rate	P/E, Fe
Vasopressor response	Vit. C

5. *Assessment of dietary intake:—*

A dietary survey may be carried out by one of the following methods:—

(i) Weighing of raw foods: The survey team visits the house-hold and weighs all food that is going to be cooked and eaten as well as that which is wasted or discarded. The duration may vary from 1 to 21 days but commonly 7 days which is called one dietary cycle.

(ii) Weighing of cooked food.

(iii) Oral questionaire method: Inquiries are made retrospectively about the nature and quantity of foods eaten during the previous 24 to 48 hours.

The data collected has to be transformed into:—

(a) Mean intake of food in terms are cereals, pulses, vegetables, fruits, milk, meat, fish and eggs.

(b) The mean intake of nutrients per adult man value or consumption unit.

6. *Vital statistics:* An analysis of vital statistics – mortality and morbidity data – will identify groups at high risk and indicate the extent of risk to community.

7. *Assessment of ecological factors:* A study of ecological factors comprises the following:—

(i) Food balance sheets: In this supplies are related to census population to derive levels of food consumption in terms of per capita supply availability.

(b) Socio-economic factors: Are like family size, occupation, income, education, customs, cultural patterns in relation to feeding practices of children.

(c) Health and educational services: PHC services, feeding and immunization programmes should also be taken into consideration.

(d) Conditioning influences: These include parasitic, bacterial and viral infections which precipitate malnutrition.

Measures to be taken at the community level to prevent malnutrition are:—

(a) *Health promotion:—*

(1) Measures directed to pregnant and lactating women (education, distribution of supplement).

(2) Promotion of breast feeding.

(3) Development of low cost weaning foods: The child should be made to more food at frequent intervals.

(4) Measures to improve family diet.

(5) Nutritional education : Promotion of correct feeding practices.

(6) Home economics.

(7) Family planning and spacing of births.

(8) Family environment.

(b) *Specific protection:—*

(1) The child's diet must contain balanced foods. Milk, eggs, fresh fruits should be given if possible.

(2) Immunization.

(3) Food fortification.

(c) *Early diagnosis and treatment:—*

(1) Periodic surveillance.

(2) Early diagnosis of any lag in growth.

(3) Early diagnosis and treatment of infections and diarrhea.

(4) Development of programmes for early rehydration of children with diarrhea.

(5) Development of supplementary feeding programmes during epidemics.

(6) Deworming of heavily infested children.

(d) *Rehabilitation*

(1) Nutritional rehabilitation services.

(2) Hospital treatment.

(3) Follow-up care.

Q.3 Enumerate:—

(a) Water borne diseases.

(b) Arthropod borne diseases

(c) Milk borne diseases

(d) Air borne diseases

Ans. (a) Water borne diseases:—

(i) Cholera.

(ii) Poliomyelitis.

(iii) Hepatitis A.

(iv) Typhoid.

(v) Hookworm infection

(vi) Amoebiasis

(b) Arthropod borne diseases:—

Ans.	Arthropod	Disease transmitted
1.	Mosquito	- Malaria - Filaria - Dengue
2.	Housefly	- Typhoid - Diarrhea - Cholera - Amoebiasis - Conjunctivitis - Trachoma
3.	Sand-fly	- Kala-azar - Oriental sore - Sand-fly fever
4.	Tsetse fly	- Sleeping sickness
5.	Louse	- Epidemic typhus - Relapsing fever - Trench fever
6.	Rat flea	- Bubonic plague - Endemic typhus
7.	Reduvild bug	- Chagas disease
8.	Hard tick	- Tick typhus - Viral encephalitis - Viral fevers

9. Soft tick   - Q fever
                   - Relapsing fever

(c) Milk borne diseases are:—

(1) Infections of animals that can be transmitted to man:—

(a) Tuberculosis.

(b) Brucellosis.

(c) Streptococcal infections.

(d) Staphylococcal enterotoxin poisoning.

(e) Salmonellosis.

(f) Q fever.

(g) Cowpox.

(h) Foot and mouth disease.

(i) Anthrax.

(j) Leptospirosis.

(k) Tick borne encephalitis.

(2) Infections primary to man that can be transmitted through milk:—

(a) Typhoid.

(b) Shigellosis.

(c) Cholera.

(d) Enteropathogenic Escherichia Coli (EEC).

Methods of pasteurization:—

(1) *Holder method:* In this process, milk is kept at 63-66° C for at least 30 minutes and then quickly cooled to 5° C. It is recommended for small communities.

(2) *HTST method:* "High temperature and short time method". Milk is rapidly heated to a temperature nearly 72° C and is hold at that temperature for not less than 15 seconds and rapidly cooled to 4° C.

(3) *UHT method:* Ultra high temperature method. Milk is rapidly heated in usually 2 stages (the second stage usually being under pressure) to between 125° C for a few seconds only. It is then rapidly cooled and bottled as quickly as possible.

(d) Air borne diseases:—

(i) Tuberculosis

(ii) Whooping cough

(iii) Diphtheria

(iv) Meningococcal meningitis

(v) Influenza

(vi) Measles

(vii) Mumps

(viii) Chickenpox

PART B

Q.4 Discuss differences between sterilization and disinfections. Discuss the role of various chemical agents in the disinfections of feces, urine and other contaminated material.

Ans. Sterilization is the process of destroying all life including spores. This is widely used in medical practice.

Disinfection is the killing of infectious agents outside the body by direct exposure to chemical or physical agents. It can refer to action of antiseptics as well as disinfectants.

Role of chemical agents in the disinfection of:—

Feces and urine: Should be collected in impervious vessels and disinfected by adding an equal volume of one of the disinfectants like:—

(i) Bleaching powder.

(ii) Crude phenol.

(iii) Cresol.

(iv) Formalin.

Then it is allowed to stand for 1-2 hours. Feces should be broken up with a stick to allow proper disinfection. If the above disinfectants are not available, an equal amount of quicklime of freshly prepared milk of lime may be added, mixed and left for 2 hours. If none is available, a bucket of boiling water may be added to the feces which is then covered and allowed to stand until cool. After disinfection, the excretal matter may be emptied into a water closet or buried in ground.

Sputum: This is best received on gauze or paper handkerchiefs and destroyed by burning. If the amount is considerable it may be disinfected by boiling or autoclaving for 20 minutes at 20 lbs pressure. Alternatively, the patient may be asked to spit in a sputum cup half filled with 5% cresol. When the cup is full, it is allowed to stand for an hour and the contents may be emptied and disposed off.

Q.5 Describe the National Immunization Schedule. Discuss the preventive and control measures of measles in detail.

Ans. In May 1974, the WHO officially launched a global immunization programme, known as the Expanded Programme on Immunization (EPI) to protect all children from six vaccine preventable diseases namely:—

(a) Diphtheria.
(b) Whooping cough.
(c) Tetanus.
(d) Polio.
(e) Tuberculosis.
(f) Measles.

The programme is now called Universal Immunization Programme.

Beneficiaries	Age	Vaccine	No. of Doses	Route of Administration
Infants	6 weeks to 9 months. 9 to 12 months	DPT Polio BCG Measles	3 3 1*	Intra muscular Oral Intra dermal Subcutaneous

Children	16 to 24 months	DPT	1**	Intra muscular
		Polio	1**	Oral
	5 to 6 years	DT	1*	Intra muscular
		Typhoid	.2	Subcutaneous
	10 years	Tetanus toxoid	1@ 1@	Intra muscular Subcutaneous
	16 years	Tetanus toxoid	1@	Intra muscular
		Typhoid	1@	Subcutaneous
Pregnant women	16 to 36 weeks	Tetanus toxoid	1@	Intra muscular

*For institutional delivery.

**Booster doses

@ 2 doses, it not vaccinated.

Cold chain: The cold chain is a system of storage and transport of vaccines at low temperature from the manufacturer to the actual vaccination site. The cold chain system is necessary because vaccine failure may occur due to a failure in storing and transporting the vaccine under strict temperature controls. The cold chain equipment consist of:—

(i) Cold box: It is meant to transport large quantities of vaccine by vehicle to out of reach sites.

(ii) Vaccine carrier: It is meant to transport small quantities of vaccine by bicycle or by foot.

(iii) Flasks: They are used if vaccine carriers are not available.

(iv) Ice-packs.

(v) Refrigerator.

Role of GMP: As the general medical practitioner is the person who is very near in a said community, therefore, he has a great role to play in the National Immunization Programme. The most important role of GMP is to create awareness among his clientele about the various diseases which can be prevented by immunization. Also, he has to motivate his patients to get immunized as early as possible.

Preventive and control measures of measles:—

Causative organism: Virus belongs to the myxovirus group, present in nasopharyngeal secretions and in blood of infected persons.

Source of infection: Nasopharyngeal secretions of the patients. No carriers.

Mode of spread:—

(i) Droplet infection.
(ii) Through fomites.

Pathology:—

Diseases more prevalent in children.

Clinical features:—

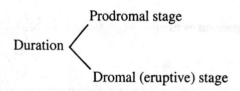

Prodromal period lasts from 2-5 days, during which there is a sudden onset of fever with catarrhal symptoms.

Diagnostic lesions during this period are the Koplick's spots which appear on the buccal mucous membrane in the form of white spots surrounded by reddish base.

Dromal (eruptive) stage begins by the 4th or 5th day when a maculopapular rash appears on the face, trunk and extremities. This gradually fades by 6th or 7th day.

Complications:—

(i) Bronchopneumonia.
(ii) Encephalitis.
(iii) Gastroenteritis.
(iv) Otitis media.

Prevention:—

Isolation of the patients and quarantine of the contacts.

The use of measles vaccination for active immunization and of immunoglobulins for prevention of infection in susceptible children. Measles vaccine is given around 9 months-1 year for effective prevention.

Q.6 Discuss the health and sanitation measures required to be taken at the forthcoming Kumbh mela.

Ans. **Sanitary measures are:—**

1. *Before the mela:—*

(a) Selection of site: The health officer and district engineer should go to the fair site for selection of site and preparation of the necessary programme for lodging houses, proper conservancy, water supply, general sanitation and the required equipment. Roads should be marked and repaired.

(b) General arrangement: All necessary materials like brooms, strings, lime and bleaching powder should be stored in godowns.

(c) Staff required and materials:—

   (i) Medical officer – one.

   (ii) Health inspector – one.

   (iii) One sweeper for every 1000 people for trench latrine.

   (iv) One sweeper for every 5000 person per day for picking up from the road.

   (v) One sweeper for every 2000 person per day for collecting rubbish and dumping it.

   (vi) Some extra sweepers dealing with other urgent matters.

   (vii) Disinfectants.

(d) Water supply: Adequate and safe water supply is of utmost important.

(e) Refuse and conservancy system: Bore hole latrines are very suitable and hygienic for the purpose. It must reach 1 feet below the sub-soil water. Dustbins, urinals and soakage pits etc. should be provided at suitable places.

2. *During the mela:—*

(a) Water Supply: Wells should be regularly disinfected. If water has been found unfit for drinking, it should be made undrinkable by pouring kerosene oil on them, or keeping a watch so that nobody drinks that unfit water. Water should be drawn by special men with proper buckets. Inspecting staff should have test tubes, potassium iodide crystals and starch powder to test the presence of chlorine and to know whether the wells have been disinfected properly or not.

(b) Refuse disposal: The refuse and road sweepings should be disposed off properly.

(c) Conservancy: Male and female latrines should be marked. They should be lighted during the night. Sweepers should be posted at each latrine for cleaning and filling the used latrine. Bleaching powder and lime should be sprinkled freely. People should be prevented from passing stool on the ground.

(d) Food sanitation: The sale of stale food, unripe and over-ripe fruits should not be permitted. One medical officer should be authorized to seize any unwholesome articles of food and destroy the same.

(e) Accommodation: There should not be over-crowding in rooms; sick people should be moved to the hospital.

(f) Medical care: Dispensaries should be under a competent medical officer. Arrangement for emergencies should be made.

PART C

Q.7 Discuss the epidemiology of rabies and role of vaccines in its prevention and control.

Ans. Rabies:—

Dog, monkey, camel and cow are all warm-blooded animals. They transmit the zoonotic disease *Rabies* to man by their bites if they are rabid.

The *causative* agent of rabies is a bullet shaped neurotropic RNA containing virus. The transfer of infection from wild life to domestic animals results in creation of urban cycle.

The *source of infection* to man is the saliva of rabid animals.

Treatment:—

There is no specific treatment for rabies, Case management includes the following procedure:—

(a) The patient should be isolated in a quiet soon protected as far as possible from stimuli such as bright light, noise or cold draughts which may precipitate spasms or convulsions.

(b) Relieve anxiety and pain by liberal use of sedatives. Morphia in doses of 30-45 mg may be given repeatedly. The drug is well tolerated and once the diagnosis is established there appears to be no reason to restrict the administration of a drug which does so much to allay acute suffering.

(c) If spastic muscular contractions are present, use drugs with curare-like action.

(d) Ensure hydration and diuresis.

(e) Intensive therapy in the form of respiratory and cardiac support may be given.

Prevention of rabies:—

1. Post-exposure prophylaxis:—

    (a) Cleansing: Immediate flushing and washing the wounds, scratches and the adjoining areas with plenty of soap and water preferably under a running tap for at least 5 minutes is of paramount importance. In case of punctured wounds catheters, should be used to irrigate the wounds.

    (b) Chemical treatment: Whatever residual virus remains in the wound after cleansing should be inactivated by irrigation with viricidal agents, either alcohol, tincture, aq. solution of iodine.

(c) Suturing: Bite wounds should not be immediately sutured to prevent additional trauma.

(d) Antirabies serum.

(e) Antibiotics and anti-tetanus serum.

(f) Observe the animal for 10 days: Observe the biting animal for at least 10 days from the day of bite. If the animal shows symptom of rabies, it should be humanely killed and its head is removed and sent for FRA test.

2. Immunization: Human anti-rabies vaccination.

Technique of administration: Ideal site for vaccination is the anterior abdominal wall, for this area offers enough space to accommodate the large quantity of vaccine to be injected. The area is divided into quadrants and a different site is used for each injection.

To ensure proper administration, a fold of skin is lifted between the thumb and other fingers with the patient in a lying down or standing position.

Q.8 List the common health problems of school children and discuss their control measures.

Ans. Health problems of school children:—

The main health problems of school children are:—

(a) Malnutrition.

(b) Infectious diseases.

(c) Intestinal parasites.

(d) Diseases of skin, eye and ear.

(e) Dental caries.

(a) *Malnutrition*: To prevent malnutrition among children mid day meal is given:—

(i) Meal should be a supplement not a substitute.//
(ii) Meal should provide 1/3rd energy, 1/2 proteins.//
(iii) Cost of meal should be low.//
(iv) Should be prepared in the school.//
(v) Locally available food should be used.//
(vi) Menu should be changed.

(b) *Infectious diseases*: Communicable disease control through immunization. A record of all immunizations should be maintained as a part of school health services.

(c) *Intestinal parasites*: Pure water should be provided to students, regular clinical examination of the child is necessary, stool examination, growth monitoring should be periodically done.

(d) *Eye health services*: Schools should be responsible for early detection of refractive errors, treatment of squint, amblyopia and detection and treatment of eye infections such as trachoma. Administration of vitamin A to children.

(e) *Dental health*: Regular dental examination. There should be inspection of teeth, cleaning which prevent gum troubles. Dental hygiene should be taught to children.

Q.9 Write short notes on:—

(a) IMR.

(b) ORS.

(c) **Population explosion.**

(d) **Vitamin A deficiency.**

Ans.(a) IMR: It is defined as the ratio of infant death registered in a given year to the total number of live births registered in the same year, usually expressed as a rate per 1000 live births.

$$IMR = \frac{\text{Number of deaths of children less than 1 year of age in a year}}{\text{Number of live births in same year}} \times 1000$$

Factors contributing to infant mortality:—

1. Biological factors:—

(a) Birth weight: A satisfactory birth weight is required for infant survival.
(b) Age of mother: Under 20 years and over 30 years mothers are at greater risk to cause infant mortality.
(c) Order of birth: Highest mortality is found among first births. The fate of the 5th child worse than the 3rd.
(d) Interval between births: The shorter the time interval between birth, greater the risk to survival of the infant.
(e) Multiple births: Infants born in multiple births face a greater risk of death.

2. Economic factors:—

Low socio-economic people have high IMR.

3. Cultural and social factors:—

(a) Breast feeding reduces IMR.

(b) Illiteracy increase IMR.

(c) Sex of child: A female child is unwelcome in the family.

(d) Broken families have high IMR.

(e) Lack of trained personals.

Prevention:—
1. Prenatal feeding: Improve the physical well being of the pregnant women.
2. Immunization: Of mother and child is very important.
3. Growth monitoring.
4. Breast feeding.
5. Family planning.
6. Efficient MCH services.
7. Improvement in the standard of living.

(b) ORS:—

The aim of ORT is to prevent dehydration and reduce mortality.

Packets of "Oral Rehydration Mixture" are now freely available at the PHC, sub-centers and hospitals. The contents of the packet are to be dissolved in one litre of drinking water. The solution should be made fresh daily and used within 24 hours. A simple mixture consisting of table salt (5g) and sugar (20 g) dissolved in 1 litre of drinking water may be safely used until a proper mixture is obtained.

The actual amount given will depend on the patient's desire to drink and by surveillance of signs of dehydration.

Older children and adults should be given as much as they want, in addition to ORS solution.

Mothers should be taught how to administer ORS solution to their children.

(a) For children under 2 years of age give a teaspoon every 1 to 2 minutes or offer frequent sips out of a cup, for older children. Adults may drink as much as they like.

(b) If the child vomits, wait for 10 minutes, then try again, giving the solution slowly, a spoonful every 2 to 3 minutes.

(c) If the child wants to drink more ORS solution than the estimated amount and does not vomit, there can be no harm in feeding him/her more.

(d) If the child is breast fed, nursing should be pursued during treatment with ORS solution.

(e) Non-breast fed infants under 6 months age should be given an additional 100-200 ml of clean water during the first four hours.

(c) Population explosion:—

Population explosion is observed under three readily observable human phenomena:—

(a) Changes in population size.

(b) Composition of the population.

(c) Distribution of population in space.

There are five processes which are continually at work within a population:—

(a) Fertility.
(b) Mortality.
(c) Marriage.
(d) Migration.
(e) Social mobility.

Population in our country is increasing at the rate of 2.1%. India has the second highest population in world.

Population of urban areas has increased due to natural growth and migration from villages because of employment opportunities, attraction of better living conditions and avaibility of social services such as education, health, transport, entertainment, etc. To reduce the population, following measures are applied:—

1. *Age at marriage:* Is increased both for males and females. Females can marry at an age of 18 and above and males at the age of 21 and above.
2. *Duration of married life:* 10 to 25% of births occur within 1-5 years of married life; 50-55% of births within 5-15 years of married life. Births after 25 years of married life are very few.
3. *Spacing of children:* Has a significant impact on the general reduction in fertility eates.
4. *Education:* Especially of girls helps in reduction of population.
5. *Economic status:* The total number of children born declines with an increase in the per capita expenditure of the household.
6. *Caste and religion:* Muslims have a higher fertility rate than Hindus.
7. *Nutrition:* All well-fed societies have low fertility rate.

8. *Family planning:* Is an important factor in fertility reduction. Health is vitally concerned with population because health in a group depends upon the:—

(i) Dynamic relationship between the number of people.

(ii) The space which they occupy.

(iii) The skill they have acquired in providing for their needs.

Hazards of population explosion are:—

1. *Food production:* It has increased in our country but population increases much faster leading to deficient or less calories per person. If food production doubles in 10 years, the population triples in 10 year.
2. *Clothing:* Against per capita, a minimum of 25 m per annum, the supply is only 14 metres.
3. *Employment* Unemployment is increasing in spite of the creation of additional jobs.
4. *Education front:* We are trying to educate every section of the society, paying special attention to children.
5. *Health programmes:* The increase in population is causing an increase in air, water and soil pollution and general ill health. Our total population ratio stands for 1:5,703 which is still far from the target. Our infant and maternal mortality rate, nutritional status, health of children are affected adversely.

(d) Vitamin A deficiency:—

The signs of vitamin A deficiency are predominantly ocular.

They include:—

(i) *Nightblindness:* Lack of vitamin A causes night blindness or inability to see in dim light. The mother herself detects it when the child is not able to see in the dark.

(ii) *Conjunctival xerosis:* This is the first clinical sign of vitamin A deficiency. The conjunctiva becomes dry and non-wettable. Instead of looking smooth and shiny it appears muddy and wrinkled.

(iii) *Bitot's spots:* These are triangular, pearly white or yellowish, foamy spots on the bulbar conjunctiva on either side of the cornea. They are usually bilateral.

(iv) *Corneal xerosis:* Cornea appears dull, dry and non-wettable and eventually opaque. It does not have a moist appearance. In more severe deficiency, there may be corneal ulceration. The ulcers may heal leaving a corneal scar which can affect vision.

(v) *Keratomalacia:* It is liquification of cornea. The cornea becomes soft and bursts open. If the eye collapses, vision is lost.

To prevent nutritional blindness:—

(a) Vitamin A prophylaxis programme: National Programme for Control of Blindness is to administer a single massive dose of an oily preparation of Vitamin A containing 200,000 IU orally to all preschool children in the community every 6 months.

(b) Fortification of foods with Vitamin A like Dalda, sugar, etc.

(c) Health education to people for primary eye care.

(d) Persuading people in general and mothers in particular, to consume generally green leafy vegetables and other Vitamin A rich foods.

(e) Promotion of breast feeding.

Q.10 Write short notes on:—

(i) Name all STDs.

(ii) F.P. measures advised to a young couple.

(iii) Sex education at school age.

(iv) Neurosis.

(v) Treatment of bed wetting in a girl of 14 years.

(vi) Problems of unmarried mother.

(vii) Social aspects of leprosy.

(viii) List vector control measures in filarial control programme.

(ix) Grades of mental retardation.

Ans. (i) Various STDs:—

Bacterial STDs:—

(a) Gonorrhea.
(b) Genital chlamydial infection.
(c) Syphilis.
(d) Chancroid.

Viral STDs:—

Genital herpes.

Genital human papilloma.

Virus infection.

Role of social factors:—

(1) *Prostitution:* A Major factor in the spread of STDs. A prostitute acts as a reservoir of infection.

(2) *Broken families:* Due to the death of one partner or due to separation. The atmosphere in such homes is unhappy and children reared in such an atmosphere are likely to go astray in search of other avenues of happiness.

(3) *Sexual disharmony:* Married people with strained relations, divorced and separated persons are often victim of STDs.

(4) *Easy money:* It provides an occupation for easy money.

(5) *Emotional immaturity:* Social factor in acquiring STDs.

(6) *Urbanization and industrialization:* These are conductive to the type of lifestyle that contributes to high levels of infection; since long working hours, relative isolation from family and geographical and social mobility foster casual sexual relationships.

(7) *Social disruption:* Caused by disasters, war and civil unrest have always increased STDs.

(8) *International level:* Travellers can import as well as export infection.

(9) *Changed behavioral pattern:* Equal rights to both sexes, independence or idea, etc.

(10) *Social stigma:* Leads to non-detection of cases, dropping out before treatment is complete.

Control of STDs:—

1. *Case detection:—*

(i) Screening of healthy volunteers: Screening of special groups, viz. pregnant women, blood donors, industrial workers, army, police, prostitutes, etc.

(ii) Contact training: It is the term used for the technique by which sexual partners of diagnosed patients are identified, located, investigated and treated.

(iii) Cluster testing: Here the patients are asked to name others persons of either sex.

2. *Case holding and treatment:* Adequate treatment of patients and their contacts. Every effort should be made to ensure complete and adequate treatment.

3. *Epidemiological treatment:* It consists of administrating full therapeutic dose of treatment to persons recently exposed to STD while awaiting the results of laboratory tests.

4. *Personal prophylaxis:—*

(i) Contraceptives.

(ii) Vaccines for hepatitis B.

5. *Health education:* Principal aim of educational intervention is to help individuals alter their behaviour in an effort to avoid STDs, that is to minimize disease acquisition and transmission.

(ii) F.P. measures advised to young couple:—

F.P. measures advised to a young couple is combined pills. The pill is given orally for 21 consecutive days beginning on the 5th day of the menstrual cycle followed by a break of 7 days during which menstruation occurs. The pill should be taken everyday at a fixed time, preferably before going to bed at night.

(iii) Sex education at school age:—

Children should be given sex education at school age by their teachers and their course should also include the sex education because of so many sexually transmitted diseases like AIDS, Syphilis, etc., Due to lack of knowledge, the students are curious towards sex and they want to experiment with it. This way they ruin there life by causing harm to their health and their careers and by the time they realize their mistakes, it is too late. Later they are guilty conscious. To prevent children from the hazards of lack of knowledge, the teachers should give them sex education so that they get familiar with it and no curiosity is left in them. They should also be taught about STD.

(iv) Neurosis: It is a mental illness characterized by irrational or depressive thoughts or behavior caused by a disorder of the nervous system usually without an organic change. The patient is unable to react normally to any life situation. He is not considered "insane" by his associates, but nevertheless he exhibits certain peculiar symptoms such as morbid fears, convulsions and obsessions.

(v) Treatment of bed wetting in a girl of 14 years:—

It can be treated by knowing the cause of it.

Heavy worm infection can cause irritation in the bladder and lead to micturition. Sometimes due to fear also the child may have nocturnal micturition. So, it is the duty to know about the fears and try to remove them from the mind. Routine stool and urine examination can give the idea of worm infection. The antiparasitic or antihelmintic drugs should be given to child.

(vi) Problems of unmarried mother:—

(a) Sexually transmitted diseases like Gonorrhea, syphilis, AIDS.

(b) Pelvic inflammating diseases.

(c) Unwanted pregnancy.

(vii) Social aspects of leprosy:—

Leprosy is the oldest disease known to man. Leprosy is often called a *"social disease"*. There are numerous social factors which favor the spread of leprosy in the community such as poverty and poverty-related circumstances eg., over-crowding, poor housing, lack of education, lock of personal hygiene and above all fear, guilt and unfounded prepdices regarding the disease. The social stigma is due to the deformity it causes. Over the centuries, a legend has grown around leprosy that it is highly contagious and that it is incurable. This has led patients to hide their early lesions and thereby delay treatment at the period when they could be most speedily cured.

(viii) List vector control measures in filarial control programme:—

Ans. *Vector control:* Mosquito Control Measures.

1. *Anti-larval measures:—*

(a) Environmental control: Reducing their breeding places. This is known as source reduction and comprises of minor engineering methods such as filling, leveling and drainage of breeding places:—
Culex: Reducing domestic and predomestic sources of breeding such as cesspools and open ditches.

Aedes: Environment should be cleaned up and got rid of water holding containers such as discarded tins, empty pots, broken bottles, etc.

Anopheles: Breeding places should be looked for and abolished by appropriate engineering measures.

Mansonia: Reduce the aquatic plants.

(b) Chemical control: Commonly used larvicides are:—

   (i) Mineral oils.

   (ii) Paris green.

   (iii) Synthetic insecticides.

Mineral oils: The application of oil to water is one of the oldest known mosquito control measures. Since the life cycle of a mosquito occupies about 8 days or so it is customary to apply oil once a week on all breeding places.

Paris green: It is a stomach poison and to be effective it must be ingested by the larvae. Anopheles are surface feeders so it is easily killed by Paris green and for bottom feeders Paris green is applied in granular formation.

Synthetic insecticides: E.g., fenthion, chlorpyrifos and abate are effective larvicides. These organophosphorus compounds hydrolyze quickly in water.

(c) Biological control: A wide range of small fish feed readily on mosquito larvae. The best known are Gambusia offense and Lebister reticulatus.

2. *Anti-adult measures:—*

(a) Residual sprays: E.g., DDT 1-2 grams of pure DDT per sq. metre are applied 3 times a year to walls and other surfaces where mosquitoes rest.

(b) Space sprays: These are those where the insecticidal formulation is sprayed into the atmosphere in the form of mist or fog to kill insects.

Common space sprays are:—

(i) Pyrethrum extract: Pyrethrum flowers form an excellent space sprays.

It has the active principle *pyrethrin* which is a nerve poison and kills the insects instantly on mere contact.

(ii) Residual insecticide: Malathion and jenitrothin.

(c) Genetic control:—

   (i) Sterile male technique.

   (ii) Cytoplasmic incompatibility.

   (iii) Chromosomal translocations.

   (iv) Sex distortion.

   (v) Gene replacement.

3. *Protection against mosquito bites:—*

(a) Mosquito net: It offers protection against mosquito bites during sleep. The net should be white to allow easy detection of mosquitoes. Best pattern is a rectangular net.

The size of opening should not exceed 0.0475 inch in diameter. The number of holes in one square inch are usually 150.

(b) Screening: Of buildings with copper or bronze gauze having 16 meshes to the inch is recommended. The aperture should not be larger than 0.0475 inch.

(c) Repellents: Like Diethyl toluamide is active against fatigans.

(ix) Grades of mental retardation.

Mental retardation may be congenital or acquired. Mental retardation is a state when psychological abilities associated with intelligence do not develop to a normal level. A child less than 75 IQ is considered mentally retarded. WHO has classified mental retardation as follows:—

(a) Profound   IQ less than 20

(b) Severe   IQ 20-35

(c) Moderate   IQ 36-51

(d) Mild   IQ 52-67

Factors affecting mental retardation in children are:—

(a) Genetic.
(b) Defective hearing.
(c) Nutritional deficiencies.
(d) Psychological deprivation during first five years of life.
(e) Birth injuries.

You must have found this book very useful in your preparation for B.H.M.S. examinations. Other titles in this series are as follows:—

1. ANATOMY
2. PHYSIOLOGY
3. PATHOLOGY
4. FORENSIC MEDICINE & TOXICOLOGY
5. PRACTICE OF MEDICINE
6. SURGERY
7. OBSTETRICS & GYNECOLOGY

B. JAIN PUBLISHERS (P) LTD.
1921, Chuna Mandi, St. 10th Paharganj, New Delhi-110 055
Ph.: 3670572, 3670430, 3683200, 3683300
Fax: 011-3610471 & 3683400
Website: www.bjainbooks.com
Email:bjain@vsnl.com

━━ SUBSCRIBE NOW ━━

THE HOMOEOPATHIC HERITAGE
(12 issues annually)
FULLY COLORED

A HOMOEOPATHIC JOURNAL WITH A DIFFERENCE

Apart from well-researched articles on Homoeopathy, each issue has regulars which include:—

- Editorial by Prof. Dr. Farokh J. Master
- Clinical Cases
- Diet and Regimen
- Famous Old Articles
- Book Review
- Homoeopathy Around the World

Chief Editor : Prof. Dr. Farokh J. Master
House Editor : Dr. Rohit Jain

For subscription details refer overleaf

B. JAIN PUBLISHERS (P) LTD.
1921, Chuna Mandi, St. 10th Paharganj, New Delhi-110 055
Ph.: 3670572, 3670430, 3683200, 3683300
Fax: 011-3610471 & 3683400
Website: www.bjainbooks.com, Email:bjain@vsnl.com

SUBSCRIPTION COUPON

Yes, I want to subscribe to The Homoeopathic Heritage.

SUBSCRIPTION RATES FOR ONE YEAR

OVERSEAS CUSTOMERS

BANGLADESH	PAKISTAN	REST OF THE WORLD
$ 18/-	$ 32/-	$ 40/-

INDIAN CUSTOMERS

INDIA	NEPAL	BHUTAN
Rs. 200/-	Rs. 200/-	Rs. 200/-

MODE OF PAYMENT

For India, Nepal & Bhutan by M.O., Bank Draft or Cheque payable at Delhi, New Delhi in favour of **B. Jain Publishers (P) Ltd.,** 1921/10, Chuna Mandi, Paharganj, Post Box 5775, New Delhi-55, India.

For Overseas by International Money Order or Bank Draft in favour of **B. Jain Publishers Overseas,** 1920, Street No. 10th, Chuna Mandi, Post Box 5775, Paharganj, New Delhi - 110 055, India.

SUBSCRIPTION ORDER FORM
(Write in Capitals)

Name ....

Complete Mailing Address ....

....

.... Pin ....

Ph. (Res.) .... Ph. (Off.) ....

E-mail ....

I am remitting Rs./US$ .... by M.O./Bank Draft/Cheque

Date ....   Signature